OPIOIDS AND POPULATION HEALTH

A PRIMER

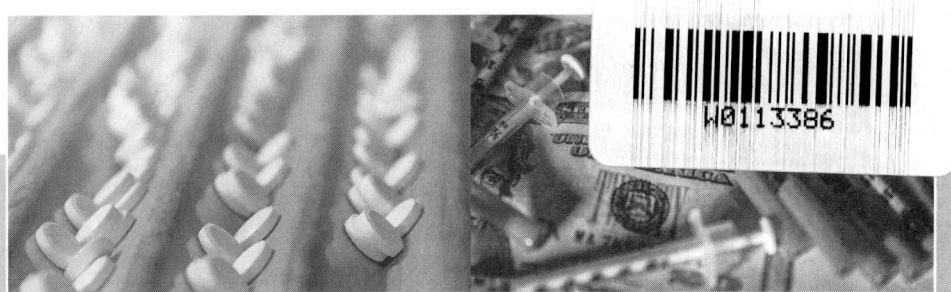

SEAN J. HALEY, PhD, MPH

Assistant Professor, Department of Health Policy and Management,
The City University of New York's Graduate School of Public Health and Health Policy

JAMES A. JOHNSON, PhD, MPA, MSc

Medical Social Scientist and Professor, School of Health Sciences,
Central Michigan University, Michigan,
Visiting Professor, St. George's University, Grenada, West Indies

LINDA J. FRAZIER, MA, RN, MCHES

Director, Addictions Initiatives, Advocates for Human Potential, Inc.
Former Chair APHA ATOD Section

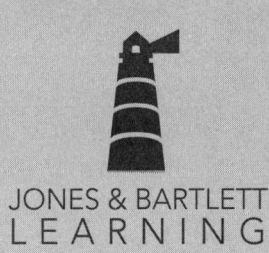

JONES & BARTLETT
LEARNING

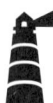

World Headquarters
Jones & Bartlett Learning
5 Wall Street
Burlington, MA 01803
978-443-5000
info@jblearning.com
www.jblearning.com

Jones & Bartlett Learning books and products are available through most bookstores and online booksellers. To contact Jones & Bartlett Learning directly, call 800-832-0034, fax 978-443-8000, or visit our website, www .jblearning.com.

22378-1

Production Credits

VP, Product Development: Christine Emerton
Director of Product Management: Laura Pagluica
Product Manager: Sophie Fleck Teague
Content Strategist: Sara Bempkins
Project Manager: Jessica deMartin
Project Specialist: David Wile
Digital Project Specialist: Rachel DiMaggio
Senior Marketing Manager: Susanne Walker
VP, Manufacturing and Inventory Control:
    Therese Connell
Product Fulfillment Manager: Wendy Kilborn

Composition: Exela Technologies
Project Management: Exela Technologies
Cover Design: Theresa Manley
Text Design: Kristin E. Parker
Media Development Editor: Faith Brosnan
Rights Specialist: Maria Leon Maimone
Cover Image (Title Page, Chapter Opener):
    © Eric Larrayadieu/Getty Images;
    © Andrew T. White/Getty Images
Printing and Binding: McNaughton & Gunn

Library of Congress Cataloging-in-Publication Data

Names: Haley, Sean J., author. | Frazier, Linda J., author. | Johnson, James A., 1954- author.
Title: Opioids and population health : a primer / Sean J. Haley, Linda J. Frazier, James A. Johnson.
Description: Burlington, MA : Jones & Bartlett Learning, [2021] | Includes
    bibliographical references and index.
Identifiers: LCCN 2020055700 | ISBN 9781284223781 (paperback)
Subjects: MESH: Analgesics, Opioid | Opioid-Related Disorders | Addiction
    Medicine–methods | Health Policy | Drug and Narcotic Control | United States
Classification: LCC RC568.O45 | NLM QV 89 | DDC 615.7/822–dc23
LC record available at https://lccn.loc.gov/2020055700

6048

Printed in the United States of America
25 24 23 22 21   10 9 8 7 6 5 4 3 2 1

Brief Contents

Contents

Foreword

In the late 20th century, the medical system in the United States repeated a mistake they had made a century before. They underestimated the risk of opioid dependence. Use of opioids increased to such an extent that an epidemic of opioid use disorder and overdose death lasting over 20 years has left no population in the United States untouched. This is a distinctly U.S. problem with rates in other countries remaining stable or increasing slightly during the same time.

The opioid epidemic provides a perfect case study of how biology, psychology, sociology, and public policy all interact to create a public health crisis. Understanding the contribution of various factors that led to the crisis is necessary for successful deployment of a public health response.

This text will help students understand the parallels of the U.S. opioid epidemic to the more typically studied outbreaks and provide the opportunity to explore how standard public health interventions might be used to address this ongoing crisis. The opioid epidemic has evolved but has not abated. While attention of the public health system has veered back toward infectious disease control and management, it is important to learn how public health principles and practices apply under different circumstances.

Working in tandem, these three authors bring together key perspectives to understanding and addressing the U.S. opioid crisis. I first met Dr. Haley while he was working as a Policy Research Scientist at the Treatment Research Institute in Philadelphia and then worked closely with him in his role as lead Evaluator for Substance Abuse and Mental Health Services Administration's (SAMHSA) launch of BHbusiness Plus—a national effort to build capacity among substance-abuse treatment providers in preparation for the Affordable Care Act. Dr. Haley's direct service background as well as his policy and management research, coupled with his national, state, and community-level experience, enable him to provide a critical overview of the political, structural, and epidemiological factors that contributed to the U.S. opioid crisis. Having worked with Linda Frazier to assess, communicate, and address the unfolding opioid crisis in Maine and across the United States between 2002 and 2015, I am familiar with her unique combination of clinical insight, thoughtful leadership, and commitment to a public health quality-improvement approach to improve access to evidence-based substance use disorder treatment. Finally, Dr. Johnson's research on health systems, along with his background in public health administration and organizational behavior, provide perspective on the necessity of collaboration across private, nonprofit, and public policy to address the ongoing opioid crisis.

Together, these authors leverage the depth of their collective experiences to bring a strong population health framework to examine how the epidemic took hold and to identify strategies to drive down opioid-related overdose mortality.

Kimberly A. Johnson, PhD, MBA, MS Ed

Dr. Johnson is Research Associate Professor in the Department of Mental Health Law and Policy at the Louis de la Parte Florida Mental Health Institute, in the College of Behavioral and Community Sciences at University of South Florida (USF). In addition to her research and teaching duties, Dr. Johnson serves as the executive director of the International Consortium of Universities for Drug Demand Reduction. Dr. Johnson earned her PhD in population health from the University of Wisconsin, Madison. Prior to her appointment at USF, Dr. Johnson was the Director of the Center for Substance Abuse Treatment within the Substance Abuse and Mental Health Services Administration (SAMHSA).

Preface

On March 18, 2020, the Director of the Centers for Disease Control and Prevention (CDC) heralded a 4% decrease in the opioid overdose mortality rate in 2018. However, the encouraging news would prove to be short-lived. By 2019, there were 70,980 drug overdose deaths in the United States, an increase of 4.6% from 2018. Seventy-one percent (50,042) of those deaths involved opioids. The following year, in the 12 months ending in May of 2020, over 81,000 drug overdose deaths occurred in the United States, the highest number of overdose deaths ever recorded in a 12-month period. It appears that fentanyl-related deaths were the driving force, up by 38% over the previous year. Although Governors across the country enforced widespread lock-downs to curtail the spread of COVID-19, it would be a mistake to think that the opioid epidemic abated as COVID-19 advanced. The uptick in overdose mortality is an indication of the fragility of our public health, healthcare, and substance use disorder treatment systems.

As states across the country responded to COVID-19, the pandemic created breaks in the opioid supply chain for both the regulated and unregulated opioid markets. It also created barriers to treatment for those receiving medication for opioid use disorders (MOUD). Both contributed to the surge in opioid overdose deaths. To their credit, in response to lockdowns, both the Substance Abuse Mental Health Services Administration and the Drug Enforcement Agency moved quickly to temporarily amend regulations to allow telehealth in lieu of in-person consultations and greater flexibility for MOUD prescribers to provide more take-home doses.

There are limited comparisons that can be made between infectious diseases and opioid use disorders. Even so, there are parallels between the COVID-19 and opioid epidemics. Both epidemics have witnessed higher rates of mortality among working class and poor communities, and both have been politicized. One example of this politization is the promulgation of the term "China virus," coined early in the pandemic to suggest that China was somehow responsible for COVID (there is credible evidence that the virus is naturally occurring and made its way from wild to domestic animals before jumping to humans). The comparison holds echoes of the rhetoric used centuries earlier to suggest that Chinese laborers were responsible for the uptake of heroin in the United States. The earlier rhetoric became part of the justification for race-based exclusion laws in the United States at the end of the 19th century.

Our country has struggled with an opioid epidemic long before COVID-19 reached our shores. According to the CDC, for over just two decades (1999–2018), almost 450,000 people died from an overdose involving any opioid. In addition to the death toll, the White House Council of Economic Advisers suggested that the cost of the opioid crisis in 2015 was $504 billion dollars. Although opioid-related mortality had started to drop, increases in overdose mortality during the

COVID-19 pandemic signals the need to continue to strengthen the substance use disorder treatment infrastructure and redouble substance use disorder and overdose prevention efforts.

Even as overdose deaths ticked upward during the COVID-19 pandemic, advances were made to counter the opioid epidemic. For example, in 2020, the U.S. Department of Justice resolved lawsuits with Purdue Pharma, brought action against 345 defendants for fraudulent opioid-related claims across 51 federal districts, and filed suit against Walmart for "fueling" the opioid epidemic.

In the wake of COVID-19, there will be opportunities to further reduce the opioid epidemic. Policymakers could strengthen the U.S. Food and Drug Administration's (FDA) regulatory authority to consider the potential population-level harms of pharmaceutical and other products. One might also consider the development of an independent watchdog entity—beyond the FDA—perhaps in the CDC, to rapidly investigate and respond to population-level harms associated with FDA-approved products. Given the staggering increases in illicitly manufactured fentanyl overdose deaths, a targeted national response is needed immediately.

On the intervention and treatment side, there is much to be done given low MOUD treatment initiation and retention rates. For example, a CDC study of approximately half of U.S. states in the first 6 months of 2019—a year before the pandemic began—found that 63% of overdose deaths had evidence of at least one potential opportunity for intervention. The recent (2020) United States Preventive Services Task Force's (USPSTF) recommendation supporting drug screening in primary care signals an opportunity to create stronger integrated care systems. The USPSTF recommendation might encourage medical associations and healthcare systems to move toward an integrated care approach where opioid use disorder treatment capability and the use of buprenorphine is not considered a specialty but rather a standard of internal medicine akin to treatment for diabetes or hypertension. In addition, SAMHSA and the Drug Enforcement Agency (DEA) might make the temporary MOUD procedural changes to assessment and medication availability initiated during COVID-19 permanent if those adaptations are found to extend treatment engagement, and reduce overdoses, hospitalizations, or deaths with minimal drug diversion. Finally, adoption of proven needle-syringe strategies to reduce infections and overdoses, providing stronger supports for former inmates with opioid-use disorder diagnoses in advance of and upon release, and establishing performance standards and measures for naloxone availability and MOUD utilization might further reduce opioid overdose mortality.

As with most diseases, political and structural factors will continue to play a role for which communities experience the greatest opioid-related losses and which are able to mount the strongest defenses. This book is intended to provide students with an overview of the biological functions of opioids; their medical use; treatment options; and the social, economic, and political structures that have contributed to the epidemic.

About the Authors

Sean J. Haley, PhD, MPH

Dr. Haley is an Assistant Professor in the Department of Health Policy and Management at the City University of New York's Graduate School of Public Health and Health Policy. Dr. Haley's research explores implementation and policy factors that influence the prevention of substance misuse and access to treatment for substance use disorders. Before completing his doctorate at Brandeis' Heller School of Social Policy and Management in 2007 where he was a NIAAA trainee, Dr. Haley held management and consultant positions in state government and not-for-profit organizations. Dr. Haley completed his post-doctorate training as a Policy Research Scientist at the Treatment Research Institute in Philadelphia where he evaluated the use of performance contracting to improve treatment initiation for patients leaving medically monitored withdrawal services (formerly known as Detox units). He served as the Senior Research Analyst for the National Association of State Alcohol and Drug Abuse Directors (NASADAD) in Washington, D.C., before joining the CUNY faculty in 2010.

Dr. Haley spent the 2018–2019 academic year on a Fulbright supported implementation study to improve alcohol screening and brief intervention in primary care within Rio de Janeiro's public healthcare system. He serves as the Immediate Past Chair for the Alcohol, Tobacco and Other Drug Section of the American Public Health Association, where he leads national efforts to reduce alcohol availability expansion efforts initiated during COVID. Most recently, Dr. Haley served as the convenor and lead facilitator of a national coalition to address racial equity and tobacco control, which produced the following value statement: "Decriminalizing Commercial Tobacco: Addressing Systemic Racism in the Enforcement of Commercial Tobacco Control." Dr. Haley completed his undergraduate degree at the University of Vermont and his MPH in policy and administration from the University of Michigan's School of Public Health.

Linda B. Frazier, MA, BS

Linda Frazier is Director of Addictions Initiatives at Advocates for Human Potential, Inc. Ms. Frazier is a registered nurse and master-certified health education specialist. Her clinical experience includes women's health, adolescent and college health, inpatient and urgent care services. Her most recent clinical role was as the outpatient behavioral health nurse responsible for assessment, monitoring, and patient education for MOUD intensive outpatient clients in treatment.

Before moving into full-time consulting, Ms. Frazier worked in a variety of leadership roles at the Harvard University Health Services and the Maine Department of Health and Human Services (DHHS) Substance Abuse and Mental Health Services (SAMHS). As Treatment Team manager and then Associate Director for SAMHS, she oversaw expansion of MOUD across Maine between 2005–2009. She served as the Maine National Treatment Network (NTN) representative and was responsible for supervision of the state opiate treatment authority (SOTA) and OTPs across the state. Since 2009, Ms. Frazier has provided training and technical assistance in behavioral health and primary care integration, process and quality improvement, and the implementation of evidence-based practices with a focus on MOUD. Ms. Frazier has served on the leadership team of the American Public Health Association (APHA) Alcohol, Tobacco, and Other Drugs Section (ATOD) since 2009. She chaired the North American Cannabis Summit (2019), which is focused on public health research, equity, policy, and best practices in state legislation and the regulatory oversight of cannabis. Her background includes teaching introduction to public health as adjunct faculty at Husson College in Bangor, Maine.

Ms. Frazier earned her BS in Adolescent Development and Health and her MA in Education from the University of Minnesota in Minneapolis. She is based in New England and travels frequently to Arizona, Taiwan, and China, where her children and partner of 35 years live and work.

James A. Johnson, PhD, MPA, MSc

James Johnson is a full professor in the School of Health Sciences at Central Michigan University, where he teaches courses in comparative health systems, organizational behavior, and health systems thinking, as well as a course in international health systems and policy.

He is a very active researcher and health science writer with over 100 journal articles and 19 books published. One book, which is read worldwide, is titled, *Comparative Health Systems: Global Perspectives*, in which he and co-researchers analyzed the health systems of 20 different countries. He is also the co-author and editor with Leiyu Shi, Johns Hopkins University, of the fourth edition of *Public Health Administration: Principles for Population-Based Management* and the recently published *Health Systems Thinking*. Eighteen of Professor Johnson's books have been selected for the permanent collection of the National Library of Medicine.

Dr. Johnson is an elected Member of the Governing Council of the American Public Health Association (APHA). He is past-editor of the American College of Healthcare Executives (ACHE) *Journal of Healthcare Management* and is currently a Contributing Editor for the *Journal of Health and Human Services Administration* and global health editor for the *Journal of Human Security and Resilience*. He works closely with the World Health Organization (WHO) in Geneva, Switzerland, and ProWorld Service Corps in Belize, Central America, on international projects and student involvement. He is a regular delegate to the World Health Congress and a member of the Global Health Council. Dr. Johnson earned his PhD at Florida State University where he specialized in health policy and organization development.

Acknowledgements

I owe a debt of gratitude to the Dean of the CUNY Graduate School of Public Health and Health Policy, Dr. Ayman El Mohandes, for recommending me to Jones & Bartlett Learning, and to my Department Chair, Dr. Terry TK Huang, for his ongoing support. I want to acknowledge the many people working in specialty care treatment centers in Delaware for their commitment to improve substance use disorder treatment and for sharing their experiences with me, as well as my colleagues in the Alcohol, Tobacco, and Other Drug Section of the American Public Health Association. I want to extend my deep appreciation to my co-authors Linda Frazier and Dr. James Johnson, and to doctoral student Ivonne Quiroz for her work on test questions and ancillary learning products. Finally, I want to thank my brother Stephen Haley and his family.

—Sean J. Haley

IN MEMORIUM

to

Elizabeth Johnson

June 19, 1989–March 29, 2014

University of Montevallo, 2013

One of far too many beautiful and talented young people taken by this epidemic

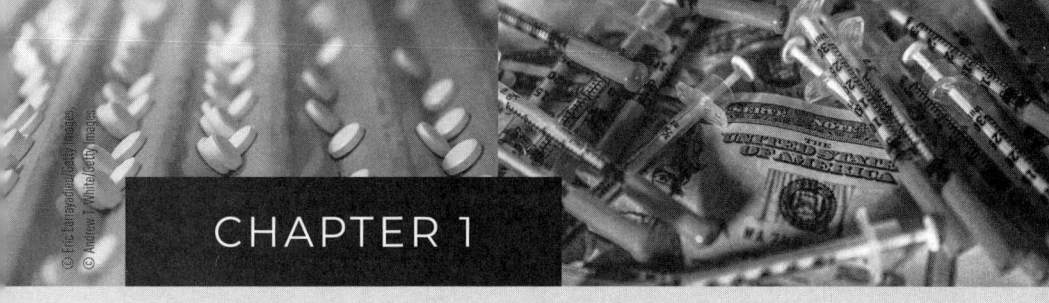

© Eric Baradat/Getty Images
© Andrew T.White/Getty Images

CHAPTER 1

What Are Opioids and How Are Opioid Use Disorders Treated?

KEY TERMS

Behavioral Therapies
Benzodiazepines
Buprenorphine
Center for Drug Evaluation and
  Research (CDER)
Chronic pain
Cocaine
Drug Enforcement Administration (DEA)
Drug Scheduling
Fentanyl
Food and Drug Administration (FDA)
Good Samaritan Law
Heroin
Illicit drugs
Medication-Assisted Therapies/
  Treatment (MAT)
Medication for Opioid Use Disorders
  (MOUD)
Methadone
Morphine
Morphine milligram equivalents (MME)

Naloxone
Naltrexone
Narcotics
Opiates
Opioid Agonist
Opioid Antagonist
Opioid Overdose
Opioid Use Disorder (OUD)
Opium
Overdose
Over the counter (OTC) medication
Partial Opioid Agonist
Population Health
Prescription Misuse
Public Health
Risk Evaluation and Mitigation Strategy
  (REMS)
Synthetic Opioids
Tolerance
Withdrawal Management

LEARNING OBJECTIVES

- Define what an opioid is
- Explain what an opioid does
- Identify the most common opioids
- Summarize the history of opioids in the United States in the 19th and 20th centuries
- Name the two different diagnostic systems used to diagnose opioid use disorders

- Differentiate opioid tolerance from opioid dependence
- Define opioid withdrawal
- Describe Naloxone and its use
- Identify the features of substance use disorder treatment
- Explain the treatment benefits of methadone and buprenorphine as medications for opioid use disorders
- Identify the strengths of behavioral (talk) therapy for opioid use disorders

To understand the opioid epidemic we must understand how the epidemic began, the complexities of opioid use disorders, and promising strategies to reverse current trends. A population approach to understanding the opioid epidemic in the United States must explore the contribution of overlapping disciplines including public health, mental health, medicine, criminal justice, market forces, and the treatment of opioid use disorders. Specifically, a population approach to the epidemic must address how some systems created to protect the public's health and safety faltered. Before we can address systems and populations, however, we must begin with understanding how opioids operate within the human body to comprehend how they have made such an indelible contribution to population level harms while serving an important role in medically supervised pain management.

Public Health and Population Health

Although we entrust local, state, and federal government officials to promulgate, monitor, and enforce protective measures, including those related to epidemics, the responsibility for public health is not limited to government entities. Public health represents the combination of scientific, policy, multi sectoral and community efforts to assure, maintain, protect, promote, and improve the health of the people (Institute of Medicine, 1988; Petersen & Lupton, 1996; Turnock, 2011). As defined by the Institute of Medicine, public health is what we as a society do collectively to assure the conditions in which people can be healthy (Institute of Medicine, 1988).

> *Public health is "what we as a society do collectively to assure the conditions in which people can be healthy"*
> **—Institute of Medicine [IOM] 1988.**

Public health has centuries'-old history of maximizing limited resources to assess health risks, create appropriate interventions, and to enforce necessary protections with attention to context. The concept of population health has an important and more recent history attributed to Kindig and Stoddart (Kindig & Stoddart, 2003). The construct has been applied to connect organizational services, especially heathcare services, to health outcomes.

Population health is "the health outcome of a group of individuals, including the distribution of such outcomes within the group."
—**Kindig and Stoddart 2003**

What Are Opioids?

Opioids include natural, semi-synthetic, and synthetic chemical compounds that attach to opioid receptors on nerve cells. Opioids include those derived from the opium plant (e.g., morphine and heroin) and synthetic opioids (e.g., fentanyl, oxycodone (OxyContin®), hydrocodone (Vicodin® and codeine) legally prescribed by medical staff for pain relief but which may be used for non-medical purposes. When individuals use prescription opioid medication for non-medical purposes, it is considered misuse and can potentially lead to dependence. Please see **Figure 1-1** for an overview of various opioids.

The term "opiates" has historically referred to natural compounds obtained from the poppy plant while "opioids" are the name given to drugs that are

Fentanyl (brand names Duragesic®, Abstral®, Ionsys®) a powerful synthetic opiate that is now being mixed with other opioids and illicit substances. A Schedule II substance, fentanyl's impact on the brain and respiratory system happens very quickly and at much lower doses. Fentanyl's potency has contributed to increasing overdose death rates since 2013 and can require multiple doses of Narcan® (naloxone) to reverse overdose and prevent death.

Heroin is derived from morphine and accessed through the unregulated market. It is a Schedule I substance designated as having no medical use.

Morphine is a Schedule II drug designated as having medical use, but also significant risk of misuse and/or dependency. It is an opiate derived from the opium poppy plants.

Oxycodone (brand names Tylox®, Percodan®, Oxycontin®) and Hydrocodone (brand name Hysingla®) are Schedule II substances. They are commercially produced semisynthetic opioids that are prescribed for the treatment of pain (acute and chronic).

Buprehorphine (brand names Belbuca®, Probuphine®, Buprenes®, Sublocade™); Methadone (brand names Diskets®, Methadone Intensol®, Methadose®, Dolophine®); Naltrexone (brand names Vivitrol®, Revia®; Naloxone (brand name Narcan®); and Suboxone® (combination buprenorphine and naltrexone) are all medications approved by the U.S. Food and Drug Administration (FDA) for the treatment of opioid use disorder. Naloxone is used to reverse opioid overdose and reduce the risk of death. These medications all occupy and act on the same opioid receptors.

Figure 1-1 Common Opioids.

synthesized by chemical processes. The term "opioids" is increasingly used as a catch-phrase for both natural and synthesized drugs. There are many types of opioids and compound combinations. The American Society of Addiction Medicine (ASAM) offers a list of brand and generic names on their website. Unless otherwise indicated, "opioids" will be used as the umbrella term for both natural and synthesized clarifies throughout this text .

Opioids are further classified as agonist, partial agonist, or antagonist according to how the drug binds to the receptors on nerve cells (Fudin, 2018). An agonist is a chemical that binds to a receptor to produce a biological response. Full agonists bind tightly to the opioid receptors and undergo significant conformational change to produce maximal effect. Partial agonists also bind to the receptor but cause less receptor activation. At low doses, both full and partial agonists may provide similar effects. However, if the dose of partial agonists increases, the analgesic (pain-relieving properties) activity will plateau and more doses will not create additional relief but may increase adverse effects (Pleuvry, 2004). Whereas an agonist causes an action, an antagonist blocks the action of the agonist, and an inverse agonist binds to the same receptor but causes an action opposite to that of the agonist.

How Long Have Opioids Been Around?

Opioids have been around for a long time. Opium has likely been in use since 2,100 BC, although the first written recording dates back to the third century BC (Norn, Kruse, & Kruse, 2005). Two millennia later in 1804, morphine was distilled from opium by E. Merck & Company in Germany (Devereaux, Mercer, & Cunningham, 2018). Morphine was widely used during the U. S. Civil War (1861–1865) to treat pain, and even then its addictive properties were recognized as "the army disease." The Merck Company would later introduce cocaine as a main ingredient in medications to treat both sinus infections and morphine addiction (Stobbe, 2017).

The next opioid innovation appeared 100 years later in 1898, when a German chemist at Bayer Pharmaceuticals discovered a British chemist's work from 14 years prior and produced diacetylmorphine, more commonly known as heroin, which was marketed to treat morphine addiction and other ailments (Hosztafi, 2001). By 1899, Bayer was producing one ton of heroin per year and selling it to 23 countries, including the United States. Producers marketed cough drops, tablets, syrups, and "potions" that contained heroin for various ailments, broadening consumption beyond Civil War veterans to everyday people (Macy, 2018). By the end of the 19th century, it was estimated that much of the population had experienced dependence, and those most affected were women and/ or came disproportionally from the upper classes (Redford & Powell, 2016). Although the alcohol temperance movement that focused on the availability and use of alcohol was well established by the end of the nineteenth century, a parallel national movement for stricter drug laws did not exist (Redford & Powell, 2016). Rather, efforts to control the use of opium initially relied on strategies to curtail the arrival of certain immigrant groups.

As China attempted to resist British imposition of an opium trade on their population, Chinese laborers arrived on the West coast in the middle of the

19th century to flee economic hardship to join the Gold Rush and then to help build the Transcontinental Railroad. As smoking opium expanded beyond work camps and grew in popularity among upper- and middle-class White circles, its public visibility would set the groundwork for racially targeted policies including, but not limited to, the Chinese Exclusion Act of 1882 (Poon, 2017). Meanwhile, pharmaceutical manufactures sold various opium products and in Boston, wealthy merchants were making sizeable profits in the opium trade (Bebinger, 2017). This is discussed in Chapter Two.

The U.S. Government began to turn its attention away from recent Chinese arrivals as the opium source and started to focus on "pharmaceutical" opium at the start of the 20th century. To counter false and exaggerated claims made about the effectiveness of products in the marketplace and to safeguard food production, the Food and Drugs Act, which established the Food and Drug Administration, was passed in 1906 (U.S. Food and Drug Administration, 2019). Among other concerns, it began to address false claims made by producers of opioid-laced tonics and syrups. Other government interventions followed including treaties and tariffs, culminating in the 1909 Smoking Opium Exclusion Act. The Smoking Opium Exclusion Act exclusively targeted opium smoking and not its use in other products, including medications (**Figure 1-2**) (Redford & Powell, 2016).

An economic approach to limit consumption took form in the Harrison Act of 1914. The Act required those involved with importing, exporting, manufacturing,

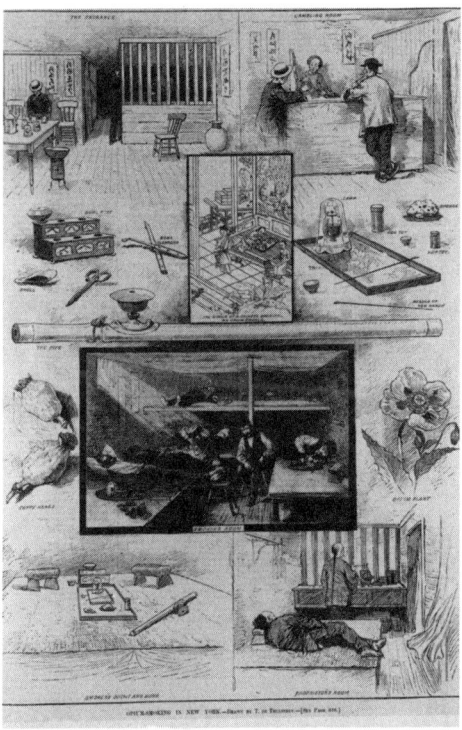

Figure 1-2 Opium Smoking in New York City.

United States National Library of Medicine. Retrieved from https://collections.nlm.nih.gov/catalog/nlm:nlmuid-101435644-img.

and distributing opium (and cocaine) to register with the Federal Government so that taxes could be levied. Part of the Act's intent was to make the products prohibitively expensive. The economic focus of the Act was not lost among public health experts who were keenly aware of the harms caused by opium and heroin and desired a more comprehensive approach.

> *Why Congress should have introduced these weak and indefinite clauses into this important measure and then dumped into the Department of Internal Revenue to interpret and enforce is not evident to those interested in this momentous question. It can possibly be explained in part by patent medicine money, in part by manufacturers and wholesalers, possibly in part by some misguided members of the medical profession both in and out of Congress* (Terry, 1915, p. 518).

The tax focus of the law allowed physicians to continue to make opium products available for a myriad of conditions, including opium addiction, since the law exempted physicians operating within their professional practice, again to the chagrin of some public health practitioners.

> *It surrounds the importer, manufacturer, wholesale and retail druggist with ample restrictions but it exempts the practising physician. Why? It has been shown repeatedly that the physician is the single greatest factor in drug addict information—worse than the patent medicine man, worse than the criminal druggist, worse than dissipation and vice!* (Terry, 1915, p. 518).

It is important to note that the Harrison Act did not do much to interfere with opioid treatment. In fact, more than 40 ambulatory treatment sites were opened in New York City and other major cities after the passage of the Act (Ghatak, 2010). However, two subsequent U.S. Supreme Court decisions (Webb v. United States and United States v. Doremus) in 1919 established that it was illegal for doctors to prescribe opioids for the purposes of maintaining an addiction, even as the decisions did not prohibit doctors from prescribing narcotics to wean a patient off of the drug (Jin Fuey Moy v. United States, 1920). Made together, these Supreme Court decisions prioritized enforcement and crime control, promoted psychopathological theories of addiction, and narrowed the scope of treatment, steering treatment away from ambulatory practices toward an increase in asylum-style treatment (Ghatak, 2010).

Following these Supreme Court decisions, in 1922, the United States enacted the Narcotic Drug Import and Export Act to regulate the importation, sale, possession, production, and consumption of narcotics other than heroin. The manufacture, importation, and possession of heroin was not made illegal in the United States until the Heroin Act of 1924 (Musto, 1999).

What Do Opioids Do?

Opioids block pain and create euphoria. The combination can create the motivation for repeated use and the opportunity for subsequent opioid use disorders. With prolonged use, tolerance to opioids develops and withdrawal symptoms may manifest if dosage is decreased or discontinued.

Table 1-1 U.S. Drug Enforcement Administration (DEA) Drug Classification

Schedule	Description	Examples
I	No medical use, high abuse potential	Heroin, LSD, Cannabis, Ecstasy, Methaqualone, Peyote
II	High abuse potential, dangerous, risk of dependence	Vicodin, Cocaine, Methadone, OxyContin, Fentanyl, Adderall, Ritalin, Methamphetamine, Dilaudid, Demerol
III	Moderate to low abuse potential, low risk of dependence	Tylenol with Codeine (less than 90 mg codeine per dose, Ketamine, Anabolic Steroids, Testosterone
IV	Low abuse potential, low risk of dependence	Xanax, Soma, Darvon, Darvocet, Valium, Ativan, Talwin, Ambien, Tramadol
V	Lower abuse potential, contain limited quantities of narcotics	Cough preparations (<200 mg./100 ml), Robitussin AC, Lomotil, Motofen, Lyrica, Parpectolin

Data from Drug Enforcement Administation. (2020). Drug scheduling. Retrieved from https://www.dea.gov/drug-scheduling

US Government Agencies

The Food and Drug Administration (FDA) is the federal agency charged with regulating food, drugs, medical devices, cosmetics, tobacco, and other products for safety (U.S. Food and Drug Administration, 2020a). The FDA Center for Drug Evaluation and Research ensures that medications are safe and effective. The FDA Center for Drug Evaluation and Research regulates over-the-counter and prescription medications, which includes biological therapies and generic drugs (U.S. Food and Drug Administration, 2020b).

The U.S. Drug Enforcement Administration (DEA), established in 1973, classifies drugs into five categories or schedules based on accepted medical use and the medication's or substance's potential for abuse or dependency. Schedule I drugs are at the highest risk of abuse or dependency and Schedule V drugs are the least harmful (see **Table 1-1**) (Drug Enforcement Administation, 2020).

Pain

Pain takes many forms. Peripheral pain is the feeling of damage to your body at the time of an injury. Central pain is the pain that accompanies a chronic injury and the body's frequent, perhaps continuous signals to the brain.

When an injury occurs, pain fibers detect the injury and transmit signals via nerve cells (neurons) through the central nervous system (along the spine to the brain). In turn, the brain releases stress-relieving hormones. These hormones—called endorphins—activate various specialized proteins called opioid receptors

(Borsodi et al., 2019). The receptors are located at the end of nerve cells in the central nervous system. When an injury occurs, or pain is present, opioids attach to the opioid receptors to block pain signals.

There are four types of opioid receptors that have been identified: mu, delta, kappa, and opioid-receptor like-1 (ORL-1) (Fudin, 2018a). Some receptors serve multiple functions.

Manufactured (human-made) opioids are chemically similar to endorphins, one of the body's natural opioids. Opioids can activate receptors because their chemical structure resembles that of the body's neurotransmitters. When a prescription or other opioids are taken, the drug uses opioid receptors that are intended for the body's endorphin hormones. However, manufactured opioids are more powerful than those that the body makes; thus they can create stronger reactions to block pain (and increase euphoria).

Research supports short-term efficacy of pharmaceutical opioids for reducing pain and improving function in non-cancer, nociceptive, and neuropathic pain lasting less than 12 weeks (Furlan, Chaparro, Irvin, & Mailis-Gagnon, 2011). Chronic pain has been defined as lasting greater that three months or beyond the time of normal tissue healing (International Association for the Study of Pain, 1986). A meta-analysis published in the *Journal of the American Medical Association* found that among patients with chronic non-cancer pain, opioid use was associated with statistically significant but small improvements in pain and physical functioning compared with placebo (Busse et al., 2018). However, it appears that initial benefits experienced from opioids may taper and exacerbate pain sensation with long-time use (National Institutes of Health, 2019; Rivat & Ballantyne, 2016).

The current opioid epidemic has resulted in federal recommendations to limit use of opioids for the management of chronic, non-acute pain. Federal and state-level guidelines for opioid prescribing have been implemented and have increased prescriber awareness of the risks of prescription opioid use (Dowell, Haegerich, & Chou, 2016). Although there are emerging advances in the development of new approaches to pain treatment, research on non-opioid pain treatments has produced limited results (Finnerup, 2019).

Euphoria

Opioids flood the brain's reward system with dopamine. Dopamine is a neurotransmitter that regulates movement, emotion, cognition, motivation, and feelings of pleasure. High levels of dopamine create overstimulation of the central nervous system, which in turn, produce the euphoric effects. Receptors activated by opioids can trigger the same biochemical brain processes associated with basic life functions that are pleasurable, such as eating, exercise, and sex.

Opioids may be prescribed to relieve pain, but opioids can also activate the reward processes described above, which can create motivation for repeated use (Kosten & George, 2002). Opioids can become addictive because they are effective at stimulating reward centers. The combination of pain reduction and euphoria (depending on administration, dose, and type of opioid) can create a powerful motivation for continued use. Once use has been prolonged, rapid deprivation of opioids can initiate physical discomfort as well as a craving for more opioids. The combination creates a strong desire to avoid uncomfortable physiological withdrawal symptoms as well as the psychological symptoms associated with cravings. Providers who treat individuals with chronic pain must balance compassionate care to manage pain with the responsibility to minimize the risk of a patient developing an opioid use disorder (Centers for Disease Control and Prevention, 2018a).

As suggested above, pain suppression and euphoria are not the only effects of opioids. As opioid molecules link to receptors in the central nervous system, they suppress the chemical processes that activate several bodily functions like wakefulness, heart rate, breathing, and alertness. Even when taken as directed, the side effects of pharmaceutical opioid use can include drowsiness, slowed respiration, and low blood pressure.

The effects of opioids vary in their duration and intensity. For example, while Alfentanil has a half-life of about 90 minutes, methadone has a half-life of between 8 to 60 hours (Oelhaf, Azadfard, & Kum, 2019). This can lead to overdose when medications are taken outside of medical supervision. In addition, since illicit drugs vary in concentration and composition, it is difficult to know their potency. For example, heroin is increasingly laced with fentanyl, which is 50–100 times more potent than morphine and can lead to overdose and death for individuals who thought they were only using heroin (Ciccarone, 2017).

Opioid Tolerance

The desire to maintain opioid use may increase with the desire to control pain, avoid withdrawal symptoms, or to re-establish euphoric sensations. In time, as the receptors become less responsive to the opioid, more of the drug is needed to achieve the same sensation. This is defined as tolerance (National Institute on Drug Abuse, 2019). Once tolerance has been created, the desire to achieve the same level of pleasure and to avoid unpleasant withdrawal symptoms can heighten motivation to continue drug use. Increases in opioid tolerance signal that central nervous system function has changed and drug dependence has begun. Scientific evidence suggests that the response to opioids can vary between patients based on genetic and other factors independent of tolerance (Oelhaf et al., 2019).

As tolerance is built, the body adjusts by increasing chemical production to activate wakefulness, breathing, and heart rate. Researchers have found that taking opioid medications for more than a few days increases risk of long-term use, which increases risk of developing an opioid use disorder (Robins, Helzer, Hesselbrock, & Wish, 2010). For example, taking pharmaceutical opioids for just five days increases the odds that a person will still be on opioids a year later (Shah, 2017). Although we cannot predict exactly who will develop an opioid use disorder, prolonged opioid use and use at higher doses creates the physiological and neurological conditions that make withdrawal difficult (National Institute on Drug Abuse, 2018c).

Opioid Dependence

Physical dependence is established when the neurons adapt to the repeated drug exposure and operate normally only when the drug is present (National Institute on Drug Abuse, 2019). The source of the opioid, whether manufactured in a pharmaceutical laboratory or derived through other processes, may have little to do with the development of dependence. **Figure 1-3** illustrates an updated label

> **WARNING: ADDICTION, ABUSE AND MISUSE; RISK EVALUATION AND MITIGATION STRATEGY (REMS); LIFE-THREATENING RESPIRATORY DEPRESSION; ACCIDENTAL INGESTION; NEONATAL OPIOID WITHDRAWAL SYNDROME; CYTOCHROME P450 3A4 INTERACTION; and RISKS FROM CONCOMITANT USE WITH BENZODIAZEPINES OR OTHER CNS DEPRESSANTS**
> *See full prescribing information for complete boxed warning.*
>
> - OXYCONTIN exposes users to risks of addiction, abuse and misuse, which can lead to overdose and death. Assess patient's risk before prescribing and monitor regularly for these behaviors and conditions. (5.1)
> - To ensure that the benefits of opioid analgesics outweigh the risks of addiction, abuse, and misuse, the Food and Drug Administration (FDA) has required a Risk Evaluation and Mitigation Strategy (REMS) for these products. (5.2)
> - Serious, life-threatening, or fatal respiratory depression may occur. Monitor closely, especially upon initiation or following a dose increase. Instruct patients to swallow OXYCONTIN tablets whole to avoid exposure to a potentially fatal dose of oxycodone. (5.3)
> - Accidental ingestion of OXYCONTIN, especially by children, can result in a fatal overdose of oxycodone. (5.3)
> - Prolonged use of OXYCONTIN during pregnancy can result in neonatal opioid withdrawal syndrome, which may be life-threatening if not recognized and treated. If prolonged opioid use is required in a pregnant woman, advise the patient of the risk of neonatal opioid withdrawal syndrome and ensure that appropriate treatment will be available. (5.4)
> - Concomitant use with CYP3A4 inhibitors (or discontinuation of CYP3A4 inducers) can result in a fatal overdose of oxycodone. (5.5, 7, 12.3)
> - Concomitant use of opioids with benzodiazepines or other central nervous system (CNS) depressants, including alcohol, may result in profound sedation, respiratory depression, coma, and death. Reserve concomitant prescribing for use in patients for whom alternative treatment options are inadequate; limit dosages and durations to the minimum required; and follow patients for signs and symptoms of respiratory depression and sedation. (5.6, 7)

Figure 1-3 Revised FDA Warning Label—September 2018.

U.S. Food and Drug Administration. (2018). *Oxycontin: Highlghts of prescribing information.* Retreived from https://www.fda.gov/media/131026/download

warning of the addictive properties of Oxycontin, first approved in 1950 (U.S. Food and Drug Administration, 2018).

As suggested, higher doses and greater frequency of use can increase the risks of developing tolerance and dependence. Physical dependence (clinically recognized in the International Classification of Diseases, Tenth Edition (ICD-10) but not in the Diagnostic and Statistical Manual of Mental Disorders, Fifth Edition (DSM-5) is often indicated when withdrawal symptoms manifest if opioids (medically prescribed or otherwise) are stopped. Symptoms of withdrawal include: increased sensitivity to pain, constipation, nausea, vomiting, sleepiness, dizziness, confusion, muscle cramping, itching, and sweating (Centers for Disease Control and Prevention, 2017). Physical tolerance, and withdrawal may be expected after prolonged opioid use, but a patient must meet additional criteria before a substance use diagnosis can be made (American Psychiatric Association, 2013; World Health Organization, 2018).

Research has suggested that there appears to be a relationship between dose and frequency such that a portion of individuals who are treated with an opioid may develop a substance use disorder (National Institute on Drug Abuse, 2019). In one study, among opioid-naïve patients who filled an opioid prescription, 5% became long-time users. The odds of long-time opioids were three times greater for patients who received between 400–799 morphine milligram equivalents (MMEs) compared with those who received less than 120 MMEs (Deyo et al., 2017). In another study, approximately 26% of patients who received frequent opioid prescriptions (4+) appeared to meet criteria for current opioid dependence (Boscarino et al., 2010).

Diagnosis of Opioid Use Disorders

There are two systems that provide criteria for the diagnosis of opioid use disorders: the *DSM-5* (5th ed.; *DSM–5*; American Psychiatric Association, 2013), and the *ICD-10*, 10th Edition (*ICD-10*, World Health Organization, 1993). The *ICD-11* is currently under review (World Health Organization, 2018).

Although generally similar, there are differences in diagnostic criteria between the *DSM-5* and the *ICD-10* (First, 2009; Saunders, 2017). The *DSM-5* is published by the American Psychological Association and is generally focused on North America. The *ICD-10* draws its authorship globally and covers medical diseases in addition to mental health and substance use disorders. It is important to understand both diagnostic criteria to facilitate a common clinical language. A diagnosis is needed to guide treatment services and is often required to obtain financial reimbursement from insurance companies. A crosswalk document that links diagnoses from the *DSM-5* to the *ICD-10* is available (Substance Abuse and Mental Health Services Administration, 2019b).

Science is moving away from the term "addiction" in favor of "substance use disorder." Indeed, the term "addict" is increasingly considered pejorative. "Addiction" does not constitute a specific diagnosis in the fifth edition of *The Diagnostic and Statistical Manual of Mental Disorders (DSM-5)*. In 2013, the categories of "substance abuse" and "substance dependence" were replaced with a single category: "substance use disorder" that contained three sub-classifications—mild, moderate, and severe. Substance use disorder symptoms fall into four major groupings: impaired control, social impairment, risky use, and pharmacological criteria (i.e., tolerance and withdrawal). The *DSM* describes a problematic pattern of use of an intoxicating substance leading to clinically significant impairment or distress with 10 or 11 diagnostic criteria (depending on the substance) occurring within a 12-month period. The American Society for Addiction Medicine has a checklist of *DSM-5* criteria for the diagnosis of an opioid use disorder that can be found on their website (American Society of Addiction Medicine, 2020).

The *ICD-10* uses similar criteria for Opioid Use Disorder, with three umbrella categories of use, abuse, and dependence. These categories include classifications of mild, moderate, or severe. The diagnosis can also be appended to indicate that the disorder is "in early or sustained remission."

Withdrawal

As tolerance grows, so does the likelihood of the body manifesting physical withdrawal symptoms in the absence of opioids. Over time, the central nervous system begins to reduce the production of select endorphins after external opioids are introduced. However, if the supply of opioids ends abruptly without tapering, the biological processes that had reduced endorphin production are no longer depressed. The resumption of endorphin production activates formerly suppressed biological processes, which can result in jitters, anxiety, muscle cramps, and diarrhea. These symptoms are part of the opioid withdrawal process, which include increased sensitivity to pain, constipation, nausea, vomiting, sleepiness, dizziness, confusion, muscle cramping, itching, and sweating (Centers for Disease Control and Prevention, 2017). Symptoms of withdrawal usually begin two to three half-lives after the last opioid dose, that is, 6 to 12 hours for short-acting opioids (heroin and morphine), and 36 to 48 hours for long-acting opioids (methadone) (Mattick & Hall, 1996). Symptoms generally peak within two to four days, and physical withdrawal generally ends between one to two weeks.

During the withdrawal process and well into the weeks and months that follow, the brains of people who have become dependent can initiate a chemical process that creates a craving for the drug. In turn, the initial cravings experienced during withdrawal may be followed by strong cravings for opioids that can last several months (Satel, Kosten, Schuckit, & Fischman, 1993). The craving process may trigger additional withdrawal symptoms (Kosten & George, 2002) and creates vulnerability for relapse. In addition, chronic stress, which is common among people who are recovering from a substance use disorder, can trigger a hormone response that is connected to the central nervous system's reward system. Once triggered, stress may chemically activate the craving process, which can create additional vulnerabilities for relapse (Sinha, 2001, 2008). Although the craving sensation may endure, in the absence of opioids, brain functioning can return to normal after a few weeks or months. Both the psychological and the physiological responses to discontinuing opioids once dependence occurs provide a powerful incentive to continue use.

Medical Management of Tapering and Withdrawal

Tapering is the processing of slowly decreasing the amount of opioid. Tapering must be done gradually with monitoring, ideally with the attention of medical professionals to avoid serious withdrawal symptoms (Centers for Disease Control and Prevention, 2019a). Although no standard opioid tapering schedule exists that is suitable for all patients, both the Centers for Disease Control and Prevention (CDC) and the FDA have formally warned providers against suddenly discontinuing opioid pain medications due to risk of serious withdrawal symptoms and related suicides (Centers for Disease Control and Prevention, 2019b; U.S. Food and Drug Administration, 2019).

Medications used in the treatment of withdrawal symptoms include opioid agonists such as methadone and buprenorphine (a partial agonist), as well as (to a lesser extent) alpha-2 adrenergic agonists such as clonidine and lofexidine (Gowing, Ali, White, & Mbewe, 2017). For decades, opioid withdrawal symptoms were largely managed with methadone because it offered high oral bioavailability, efficacy, long duration symptom relief, and affordability (Kleber & Riordan, 1982). Strict government controls to monitor access and distribution plus ambivalence to using a medication that created dependence to treat dependence led to the development and use of buprenorphine to manage withdrawal symptoms. Buprenorphine-supported withdrawal appears superior to clonidine (Ling et al., 2005).

The most effective withdrawal management method is to initiate a medication (described in the treatment section below as medication for opioid used disorders (MOUD); methadone or buprenorphine) for the opioid rather than focusing on complete withdrawal to initiate treatment (O'Connor, 2005; Stein & Friedmann, 2007). The goal of medication induction before withdrawal begins is to suppress opioid withdrawal as rapidly as possible and to initiate treatment. The goal of medication management is to use medication to prevent the emergence of opioid withdrawal symptoms, suppress cravings for opioids, and reduce the effect of self-administered opioids should a patient decide to supplement opioid intake.

The initiation of buprenorphine to manage withdrawal is often preferred. Unlike methadone, buprenorphine is a partial agonist. Partial agonists bind to and activate a receptor but are not able to elicit the total response that is created by full agonists (e.g., heroin, methadone, and oxycodone). However, in the presence of a full agonist, buprenorphine acts as an antagonist, competing with the full agonist for the same receptor, thereby blocking the full agonist from producing its maximum effect. There appears to be no difference between buprenorphine and methadone for successful induction to treatment, although buprenorphine withdrawal management may be associated with higher rates of treatment engagement (Gowing et al., 2017).

Following concerns raised by the World Health Organization (2009b) about the need to clarify medical responsibilities, the term "detoxification" is being replaced with "withdrawal management" (American Society of Addiction Medicine, 2014; Comer et al., 2015).

"The liver performs detoxification and clinicians manage withdrawal symptoms."
—American Society of Addiction Medicine (ASAM) (2015)

Withdrawal management often relies on medication to reduce the severity of opioid withdrawal symptoms. Symptom severity is associated with the type of opioid (short-acting yields more intense withdrawal); amount used; duration of use; and setting factors (Kleber, 2007).

Complete withdrawal is rarely needed to initiate MOUD. Withdrawal management centers (sometimes still called "detoxification centers") are typically affiliated with hospitals or stand-alone substance use disorder treatment programs.

The goals of managing opioid withdrawal symptoms in a continuing care system are to (1) safely manage physical symptoms of withdrawal and (2) motivate and engage the patient into some form of continued substance use disorder treatment (McLellan & Meyers, 2004). An individual's motivation to initiate full opioid withdrawal can vary from a desire to abstain from opioids and not use MOUD (e.g. methadone or buprenorphine) to support treatment and recovery, to wanting to reduce tolerance to cheapen the costs of future drug use (Diaper, Law, & Melichar, 2014). Those who have initiated MOUD can later initiate medically supervised withdrawal if they no longer want to continue with medication (Sigmon et al., 2012).

Withdrawal management can provide a pathway to treatment initiation, but it is not treatment (R. P. Mattick & Hall, 1996), and relapse rates are exceptionally high (Smyth, Barry, Keenan, & Ducray, 2010). Up to 70% of patients from inpatient medically managed services who experience complete withdrawal do not transition to specialty care treatment (Chutuape, Jasinski, Fingerhood, & Stitzer, 2001; Haley, Dugosh, & Lynch, 2011; Mark, Dilonardo, Chalk, & Coffey, 2002). Patient vulnerability immediately after withdrawal management that is not connected to MOUD or to other services leaves patients susceptible to relapse and overdose (Davison et al., 2006; Strang et al., 2003).

Overdose Reversal

As discussed, synthetic and organic opioids activate the brain's opioid receptors, which regulate breathing and influence an individual's experience of pain and euphoria. Taking too much of an opioid, known as an overdose, can cause fatal respiratory depression. During respiratory depression, breathing slows below the level required to effectively transfer oxygen to the vital organs. As oxygen saturation (normally greater than 97%) falls below 86%, brain function slows; the individual becomes unresponsive; and the heart rate decreases, which leads to cardiac arrest and death (World Health Organization, 2013). Three core opioid overdose symptoms include: pinpoint pupils, unconsciousness, and respiratory depression (World Health Organization, 2013).

Naloxone is a powerful µ opiate antagonist that reverses opiate-induced respiratory depression. Naloxone has a stronger affinity to opioid receptors than many other opioids so it replaces them at the receptor sites for a limited time. The replacement can reverse an overdose, rapidly reversing respiratory depression to allow a person to breathe normally within two to eight minutes. Although naloxone medication remains effective for about two hours, medical assistance should be summoned immediately as the type and amount of opioid in the body can influence naloxone's effectiveness (National Institute on Drug Abuse, 2017; Centers for Disease Control and Prevention, 2018b). For example, highly potent opioids (e.g., fentanyl) or large quantities of opioids may require multiple doses of naloxone to maintain respiratory function (National Institute on Drug Abuse, 2017).

Naloxone rescue kits come in a variety of formulations and administration methodologies (Kerensky & Walley, 2017). Most states have passed some version of a Naloxone Access Law, which authorizes first responders to administer an "opioid antagonist" and protects them from civil and criminal liability (Rees, Sabia, Argys, Latshaw, & Dave, 2017). Many states have also passed a "Good Samaritan Law," which protects bystanders who in good faith seek medical assistance for someone experiencing a drug-related overdose (Rees et al., 2017). Both community-based opioid overdose prevention/naloxone distribution programs and hospital emergency department naloxone distribution programs have proven effective in reducing opioid-related overdose deaths (Clark, Wilder, & Winstanley, 2014; McDonald & Strang, 2016). Although the FDA has recommended that medical providers co-prescribe naloxone with an opioid (U.S. Food and Drug Administration, 2018), the CDC has noted that too little naloxone is being made available in the areas that need it the most (Centers for Disease Control and Prevention, 2019c).

High doses of naloxone can initiate acute withdrawal symptoms. Those experiencing precipitated withdrawal initiated by naloxone will experience intense cravings to use opioids (Kerensky & Walley, 2017). In turn, naloxone overdose survivors rarely seek opioid treatment. Stronger linkages between naloxone administration and treatment initiation may be warranted since starting a patient on a long-acting agonist (buprenorphine) after an overdose event has been associated with less self-reported opioid use and reduced utilization of inpatient services at 30 days (D'Onofrio et al., 2015).

Treatment for Opioid Use Disorders

"A common misperception is that addiction is a choice or moral problem, and all you have to do is stop. But nothing could be further from the truth....The brain actually changes with addiction, and it takes a good deal of work to get it back to its normal state. The more drugs or alcohol you've taken, the more disruptive it is to the brain."

Dr. George Koob, Director of National Institute on Alcohol Abuse and Alcoholism (as cited in Wein, 2015, p. 1)

In a landmark study, McClellan et al., compared the genetic heritability and relapse rates among substance use disorders and three common medical conditions: hypertension, diabetes mellitus, and asthma (McLellan, Lewis, O'Brien, & Kleber, 2000). The authors found comparable relapse and heritability rates across conditions, suggesting that substance use disorders are like chronic conditions that require multiple interventions, ongoing monitoring, and support (McLellan, Arndt, Metzger, Woody, & O'Brien, 1993). The study highlighted that relapse happens across conditions (e.g., substance use disorders, diabetes, hypertension and asthma), suggesting that moral characterizations of substance use disorders were unfounded.

The treatment of opioid use disorders helps individuals regain health. Treatment can occur in a variety of settings. Treatment uses behavioral, and pharmacotherapy interventions, or a combination of these (See **Figue 1-4**).

ASAM has developed a treatment continuum consisting of four broad levels of service that range from early intervention (level 1) to medically managed intensive inpatient services (level 4) (Mee-Lee, 2013). Decimal numbers are used

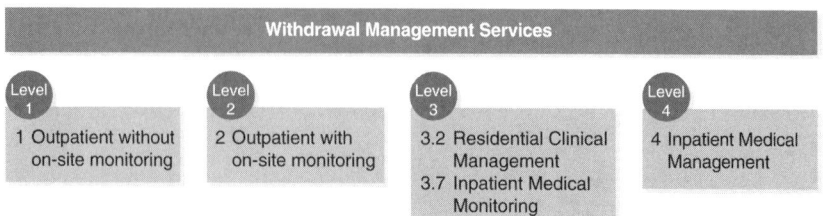

Figure 1-4 Withdrawal Management Levels of Care.
Data from Mee-Lee, D. (Ed.). (2013). *The ASAM criteria*. Chevy Chase, MD: American Society of Addiction Medicine.

within these four levels to express gradations of intensity of services. The ASAM criteria includes five levels of withdrawal management services that correspond to ASAM's treatment levels. The services may be provided separately from or concurrently with the aforementioned level-of-care services, by the same clinical staff, and in the same treatment setting (Medicaid Innovation Accelerator Program, 2017).

Treatment duration varies based on patients' needs and the type of treatment, although 12 months is considered the minimum for medication maintenance for opioid use disorders (Cornish, Macleod, Strang, Vickerman, & Hickman, 2010). Patients may transition between levels of care and intensity of services as symptoms diminish and return (Zhang, Friedmann, & Gerstein, 2003).

Medication for Opioid Use Disorders (MOUD)

MOUD (sometimes known as Medication Assisted Treatment or MAT) is the use of medications like methadone and buprenorphine (often used with behavioral therapies) to treat substance use disorders (National Institute on Drug Abuse, 2018a). Research shows that a combination of medication and behavioral therapies can successfully treat opioid disorders (Schuckit, 2016). The prescribed medication operates to normalize brain chemistry, block the euphoric effects of opioids, relieve physiological cravings, and normalize body functions without the negative effects of the illicit opioid (Schuckit, 2016).

A common misconception associated with MOUD is that it substitutes one drug for another. The concern is understandable. People recovering from an opioid use disorder often describe feeling as though they were under the control of the drug and are concerned about trading one external agent for another (Murphy & Irwin, 1992). The intent of MOUD medications to relieve the withdrawal symptoms and psychological cravings that cause chemical imbalances in the body. MOUD therapies provide a safe and controlled level of medication to overcome the use of an abused opioid. There is no maximum recommended duration of maintenance treatment, and for some patients, treatment may continue indefinitely. All treatment should be guided by a treatment plan, developed between the provider and the patient. Treatment plans should include the type(s) of treatment, dose, expected duration, and a regular check-in procedure to assess the patient's well-being. While there has been some suggestion that behavioral therapies may not offer added value in addition to MOUD (Amato, Minozzi, Davoli, & Vecchi, 2011), behavioral therapy alone, without the support of MOUD, is <u>not</u> recommended (Mattick, Breen, Kimber, & Davoli, 2009; Schuckit, 2016).

Unfortunately, publicly funded substance abuse treatment programs appear to lag behind privately funded centers in their delivery of evidence-based treatments, including MOUD (Abraham, Knudsen, Rieckmann, Roman, & Drugs, 2013; Knudsen &. Roman, 2012). ASAM has published guidelines for the use of medications to treat opioid use disorders (American Society of Addiction Medicine, 2015). Randomized controlled studies have found a range of retention for medication-only treatment (37%–98%) at 12 months (Timko, Schultz, Cucciare, Vittorio, & Garrison-Diehn, 2016). Methadone receipt was associated with longer retention rates at four and six months than buprenorphine (Timko et al., 2016). Methadone, buprenorphine, and naltrexone are the medications most commonly used to treat opioid abuse. A description of each medication follows. See **Table 1-2**.

Methadone is a synthetic opioid agonist that has been used successfully since the 1950s to treat opioid use disorders (World Health Organization, 2009a). As a full agonist, methadone occupies the same receptors but at a slower rate than other medications (allowing it to last longer than naltrexone or buprenorphine). Methadone is offered as a pill, liquid, or wafer and is taken once a day. Methadone causes dependence, but—because of its steadier influence on the μ opioid receptors—it produces minimal tolerance and euphoria while alleviating craving (Kosten & George, 2002).

Methadone treatment in the United States is offered through specialized opioid treatment programs (OTPs). OTPs provide MOUD for people diagnosed with an opioid-use disorder. OTPs operate under strict operational guidelines for

---

Table 1-2 **FDA-Approved Products for the Treatment of Opioid Dependence**

Buprenorphine:

- Bunavail (buprenorphine and naloxone) buccal film
- Cassipa (buprenorphine and naloxone) sublingual film
- Probuphine (buprenorphine) implant for subdermal administration
- Sublocade (buprenorphine extended-release) injection for subcutaneous use
- Suboxone (buprenorphine and naloxone) sublingual film for sublingual or buccal use, or sublingual tablet.
- Subutex (buprenorphine) sublingual tablet
- Zubsolv (buprenorphine and naloxone) sublingual tablets

Methadone:

- Dolophine (methadone hydrochloride) tablets
- Methadose (methadone hydrochloride) oral concentrate

Naltrexone:

- Vivitrol (naltrexone for extended-release injectable suspension) intramuscular

U.S. Food & Drug Administration. (n.d.). Information about medication assisted treatment (MAT). Retrieved from https://www.fda.gov/drugs/information-drug-class/information-about-medication-assisted-treatment-mat

patient eligibility, dosing, and diversion safeguards under federal scrutiny from the Substance Abuse Mental Health Services Administration (SAMHSA) and the DEA (Substance Abuse Mental Health Services Administration, 2015). Qualifying OTPs with certified medical providers can also offer buprenorphine.

Patients are generally started on a daily methadone dose of 20 mg to 30 mg, with increases of 5 mg to 10 mg until a dose of 60 mg to 100 mg per day is achieved, depending on the patient's history of opioid use. Doses that produce full suppression of opioid craving have been found to be more effective at retaining patients in therapy (Faggiano, Vigna-Taglianti, Versino, & Lemma, 2003). Patients' needs vary; some patients can be maintained at lower levels while others require higher levels than guidelines suggest (Trafton, Minkel, & Humphreys, 2006). Patients tend to stay on methadone for 6 months to 3 years. Relapse is common among patients who discontinue methadone too soon, and many patients have benefited from lifelong methadone maintenance.

Buprenorphine, approved by the FDA in 2002, is a partial agonist that has strong binding abilities. It readily replaces other opioids, does not cause pleasurable effects and effectively stops withdrawal symptoms (National Institute on Drug Abuse, 2018b; Substance Abuse and Mental Health Services Administration, 2019a). Buprenorphine has a longer half-life than methadone, which allows it to be prescribed for dosing on alternate days or three times per week. Buprenorphine treatment recommendations have changed considerably since 2002 (Martin, 2018). The usual maintenance dose of buprenorphine is 16 to 24 mg/day (although some patients are comfortable at 8 to 12 mg and others need 24 to 32 mg) (Ang-Lee et al., 2006; Hopper, Wu, Martus, & Pierre, 2005). A comprehensive literature review and analysis have concluded that buprenorphine is equivalent to methadone in medium and high doses (Mattick, Breen, Kimber, & Davoli, 2014).

Before 2021, Buprenorphine was prescribed or dispensed in physician offices by certified physicians, until 2016 when eligibility expanded to include physicians' assistants, and nurse practitioners, significantly increasing treatment access (National Institute on Drug Abuse, 2018b). In October 2002, the FDA approved two buprenorphine products (Suboxone® and Subutex®) for the treatment of opioid use disorders. As buprenorphine prescribers have expanded however, practice patterns have not kept pace with emerging science. Findings across 7 areas: location of buprenorphine induction, combining buprenorphine with a benzodiazepine, relapse during buprenorphine treatment, requirements for counseling, uses of drug testing, use of other substances during buprenorphine treatment, and duration of buprenorphine treatment merit review by prescribers (Martin, Chiodo, Bosse, & Wilson, 2018). Until 2021, medical providers seeking to prescribe buprenorphine for any number of patients were required to complete an 8 hour training and secured a waiver (Substance Abuse and Mental Health Services Administration, 2019a). Following legislation in 2006, physicians may treat up to 275 patients with buprenorphine (Substance Abuse and Mental Health Services Administration, 2019c). Legislation passed in 2016 expanded prescribing privileges and allowed physician assistants and nurse practitioners to treat up to 30 patients once certified. Although availability appears to be improving with the expansion of eligible treatment providers and caseloads (Knudsen et al., 2017), considerable barriers remain (Hutchinson, Catlin, Andrilla, Baldwin, & Rosenblatt, 2014;

Table 1-3 Buprenorphine Care: Previous Approaches Compared with New Findings and Recommendations

---

Seven Areas of Research Supported Modifications to Buprenorphine Clinical Practice

- Induction practices that increase timely access and continuity of care
- Relapse responses that address needs and continue treatment engagement
- Counseling and support services as needed
- Drug testing with the goal of addressing relapse
- Patient centered responses to the use of other substances during treatment – including benzodiazepines
- Duration of buprenorphine treatment based on client perceptions of risk or benefit

Reproduced from Martin, S. A., Chiodo, L. M., Bosse, J. D., & Wilson, A. (2018). The next stage of buprenorphine care for opioid use disorder. *Annals of Internal Medicine, 169*(9), 628–635. doi:10.7326/m18-1652

Knudsen & Roman, 2012). Recognizing that the training requirement was created an access barrier, on January 14, 2021 the U.S. Department of Health and Human Services announced publication of *Practice Guidelines for the Administration of Buprenorphine for Treating Opioid Use Disorder* for the purpose of expanding access to buprenorphine for MOUD treatment. This guideline creates an exception to certification requirements for physicians to treat up to 30 patients in their practice with buprenorphine (U.S. Department of Health and Human Services, 2021). A summary of changes to buprenorphine recommendations appears in **Table 1-3** (Martin, Chiodo, Bosse, & Wilson, 2018).

Like methadone and buprenorphine, naltrexone is used to help patients avoid relapse after they have been detoxified from opioid dependence. As an antagonist, its main therapeutic action is to monopolize μ opioid receptors in the brain so that addictive opioids cannot link up with them and stimulate the brain's reward system. Naltrexone is a non-addictive μ opioid receptor antagonist administered at 50 mg per day, up to 200 mg twice weekly, or as an intramuscular injection that lasts for 30 days. Naltrexone has demonstrated similar effectiveness to buprenorphine for maintaining short-term opioid abstinence (Minozzi et al., 2011; Tanum et al., 2017).

Behavioral Therapies

Behavioral therapies can help motivate people to participate in drug treatment, offer strategies for coping with drug cravings, teach ways to avoid drugs and prevent relapse, and help individuals deal with relapse if it occurs. Behavioral therapies can also help people improve communication, relationships, and parenting skills, as well as family dynamics. Current research is constrained in its ability to offer guidance on the types or levels of psychosocial services that should be provided for which substance use disorders, or on how to adapt psychosocial supports across clinical settings or patient groups (Office of The Assistant Secretary for Planning and Evaluation, 2019).

Under current federal law, patients receiving treatment from an OTP must receive counseling, which could include different forms of behavioral therapy (Substance Abuse and Mental Health Services Administration, 2020). Behavioral therapy can be either focused on the individual, on group therapies with a well-trained counselor, or a combination of both. Group therapy can allow those in treatment to create new social bonds and provide positive reinforcement, and help enforce behavioral patterns that focus on ways of living without substance use. Some of the more established behavioral treatments for opioid use disorders include: contingency management, cognitive-behavioral therapy, motivational interviewing, and risk reduction counseling. A meta-analysis found limited added benefit for behavioral therapies when combined with methadone maintenance therapies (Amato et al., 2011), but a subsequent review appears to suggest added benefits (Dugosh et al., 2016).

Contingency Management

Contingency management delivers tangible rewards to patients to reinforce positive behaviors such as abstinence (Petry, 2000). Begun in the late 1960s (Tighe & Elliott, 1968), the treatment provides vouchers to patients who meet pre-determined thresholds. The vouchers are redeemable for retail items or financial incentives (Davis et al., 2016). Contingency management interventions have been shown to improve opioid abstinence and retention rates, and like other interventions, results decay once treatment ends (Davis et al., 2016).

Compared with methadone-only patients, patients receiving methadone with contingency management were more likely to be retained at three and six months (Timko et al., 2016). Retention rates for MOUD (without behavioral therapy) at two years is 38% (Timko et al., 2019) but the addition of behavioral therapies can improve retention to 53% (Dutra et al., 2008).

Community Reinforcement Approach (CRA)

Community Reinforcement Approach (CRA) is an intensive 24-week outpatient therapy. Begun in the 1970s (Hunt, Azrin, & therapy, 1973), the goal is to help patients adopt behaviors that are more rewarding than using drugs. CRA therapy includes several procedures (Meyers, Roozen, Smith, & Health, 2011):

1. Functional analysis of substance use—explores antecedents and positive and negative consequences of substance use
2. Sobriety sampling—patient agreement for a time-limited abstinence
3. Treatment plan—includes several inventories, including one related to happiness and assignments
4. Behavioral skills training to assist with problem solving, communication, etc.
5. Job skills training
6. Social and recreational counseling—provide alternatives to usual routine

An additional contingency management component has been added that seems to enhance treatment effects for opioid-use disorders (Bickel, Amass, Higgins, Badger, & Esch, 1997).

12-Step Facilitation

Twelve-step facilitated peer programs (Narcotics Anonymous) remain popular. The goal of 12-step facilitation is to help the patient engage in 12-step self-help groups, thereby promoting abstinence. At their core, 12-step programs focus on:

1. Acceptance; acknowledging that drug addiction is a chronic, progressive disease; and that willpower alone is insufficient to overcome the problem,
2. Surrender, which involves giving oneself over to a higher power and accepting support structure of other recovering addicted individuals
3. Active involvement in 12-step meetings and related activities

Lastly, findings related to cognitive behavioral therapy plus MOUD are inconsistent but may offer benefit for prescription drug misuse (Fiellin et al., 2013; Moore et al., 2016). In addition, although ongoing treatment and support is widely acknowledged to be a critical component of any treatment plan (National Institute on Drug Abuse, 2018b), additional research evidence for 12-step programs would be helpful (Ferri, Amato, & Davoli, 2006). The inclusion of other support services in treatment planning and delivery, including legal and housing services, improves patients' recovery efforts (National Institute on Drug Abuse, 2018b). See **Figure 1-5**.

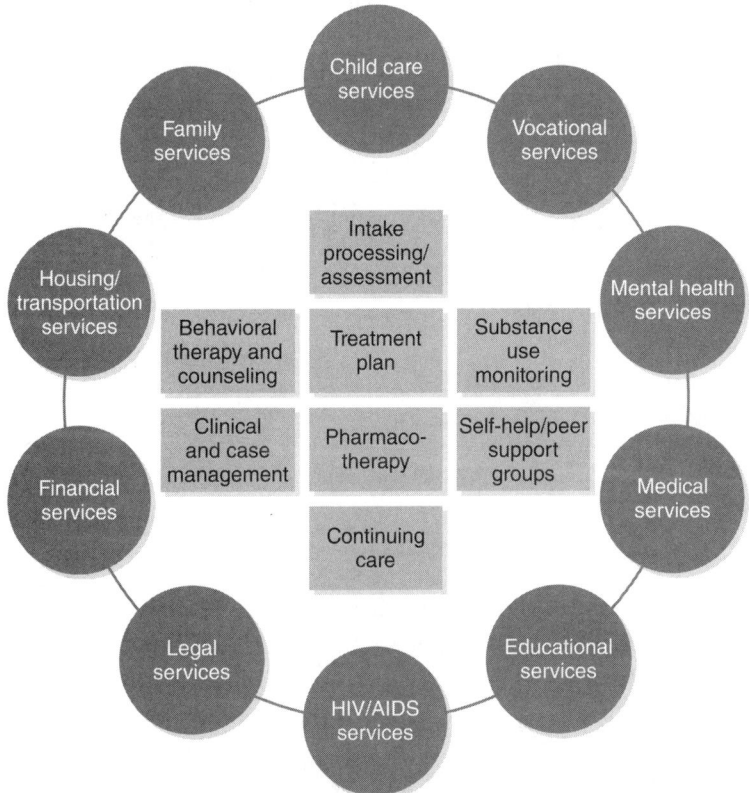

Figure 1-5 Components of Comprehensive Drug Abuse Treatment.

Treatment Is Effective but Underutilized

A 2020 National Academies of Sciences, Engineering, and Medicine report reviewed the literature on MOUD and found that most people who could benefit from this treatment did not receive medication and that access was inequitable across population subgroups and treatment settings (Mancher & Leshner, 2019). Of the approximately 2 million people with an opioid use disorder in 2018, only 10% received treatment. Among those with a substance use disorder, the vast majority (95%) did not perceive a need for treatment (Substance Abuse and Mental Health Services Administration, 2019b).

There are many barriers to opioid treatment. Despite the availability of publicly supported treatment programs, only 36% of specialty treatment programs offered at least one medication for opioid use disorder treatment in 2017 (Abraham et al., 2020), and just a small fraction of patients who receive treatment actually receive medication (Knudsen, 2010). Historically, treatment availability for people who inject drugs has been low with mean drug treatment coverage remaining close to 6% (persons who inject drugs in treatment/persons who inject drugs within a metropolitan statistical area) between 1993 and 2007 (Tempalski, Cleland, Williams, Cooper, & Friedman, 2018). Although insurance coverage increased from 44% to 68% for mental health disorders between 1986 and 2014, coverage remained stable for substance use at approximately 45% (Mark et al., 2016). In addition, publicly funded specialty care substance abuse treatment services often suffer from shortages in qualified staff and funding (Alagoz, Hartje, & Fitzgerald, 2017; Jones, Campopiano, Baldwin, & McCance-Katz, 2015). More recent research and discussion has begun to turn to identifying barriers and strategies to improve access to medical treatment for opioid use disorders (Madras, Ahmad, Wen, & Sharfstein, 2020). Improving access to opioid treatment is critical as treatment availability has been associated with lower opioid related mortality (Haley, Maroko, Wyka, & Baker, 2019).

Discussion Questions

1. Are there any "good" opioids? Explain.
2. Why does the government (DEA) assign various drugs and drug formulation to different schedules?
3. What were some of the first uses of opioids in the United States?
4. Do you think opioid dependence was a problem in the 19th and 20th centuries?
5. If it was a problem then, why do you think it has become a problem again?
6. Are opioid use disorders more like chronic diseases or acute medical conditions?
7. Why do you think people become dependent on opioids and find it hard to stop using them?

8. Do you think that people who develop an opioid use disorder are perceived poorly or face stigma? If yes, explain why. If no, explain why not.
9. Why is the treatment of opioid use disorders more successful with medication than behavioral therapies?
10. Evaluate why opioid use disorder treatment is underutilized using:
    a. A structural analysis
    b. Health systems (institutional payment and organization) analysis
    c. Individual motivational (beliefs and behaviors) analysis

References

Abraham, A. J., Andrews, C. M., Harris, S. J., & Friedmann, P. D. (2020). Availability of medications for the treatment of alcohol and opioid use disorder in the USA. Neurotherapeutics, 1–15.

Abraham, A. J., Knudsen, H. K., Rieckmann, T., & Roman, P. M. (2013). Disparities in access to physicians and medications for the treatment of substance use disorders between publicly and privately funded treatment programs in the United States. *Journal of Studies on Alcohol and Drugs, 74*(2), 258–265.

Alagoz, E., Hartje, J., & Fitzgerald, M., (2017). National Workforce Report. Available: https://www.drugsandalcohol.ie/28384/1/ATTC_Network_Natl_Report2017.pdf

Amato, L., Minozzi, S., Davoli, M., & Vecchi, S. (2011). Psychosocial combined with agonist maintenance treatments versus agonist maintenance treatments alone for treatment of opioid dependence. *Cochrane Database of Systematic Reviews*, (10), CD004147.

American Psychiatric Association. (2013). *Diagnostic and statistical manual of mental disorders* (5th ed.). American Psychiatric Publishing.

American Society of Addiction Medicine. (2014). The ASAM performance measures for the addiction specialist physician. In: *American Society for Addiction Medicine*. Chevy Chase, Maryland.

American Society of Addiction Medicine. (2015). *National practice guideline for the use of medications in the treatment of addiction involving opioid use*. Retrieved from https://www.asam.org/docs/default-source/practice-support/guidelines-and-consensus-docs/asam-national-practice-guideline-supplement.pdf.

American Society of Addiction Medicine. (2020). *DSM-5 criteria for diagnosis of opioid use disorder.* Retrieved from https://www.asam.org/docs/default-source/education-docs/dsm-5-dx-oud-8-28-2017.pdf?sfvrsn=70540c2_2

Ang-Lee, K., Oreskovich, M. R., Saxon, A. J., Jaffe, C., Meredith, C., Ellis, M. L. K., . . . Knox, P. C. (2006). Single dose of 24 milligrams of buprenorphine for heroin detoxification: An open-label study of five inpatients. *Journal of Psychoactive Drugs, 38*(4), 505–512.

Banta-Green, C. J., Maynard, C., Koepsell, T. D., Wells, E. A., & Donovan, D. M. (2009). Retention in methadone maintenance drug treatment for prescription-type opioid primary users compared to heroin users. *Addiction, 104*(5), 775–783. doi:10.1111/j.1360-0443.2009.02538.x

Bickel, W. K., Amass, L., Higgins, S. T., Badger, G. J., & Esch, R. A. (1997). Effects of adding behavioral treatment to opioid detoxification with buprenorphine. *Journal of Consulting and Clinical Psychology , 65*(5), 803–810. doi:10.1037/0022-006x.65.5.803

Borsodi, A., Bruchas, M., Caló, G., Chavkin, C., Christie, M. J., Civelli, O., . . . Zimmer, A. (2019). Opioid receptors (version 2019.4) in the IUPHAR/BPS Guide to Pharmacology Database. *IUPHAR/BPS Guide to Pharmacology CITE, 2019*(4).

Boscarino, J. A., Rukstalis, M., Hoffman, S. N., Han, J. J., Erlich, P. M., Gerhard, G. S., & Stewart, W. F. (2010). Risk factors for drug dependence among out-patients on opioid therapy in a large US health-care system. *Addiction, 105*(10), 1776–1782.

Busse, J. W., Wang, L., Kamaleldin, M., Craigie, S., Riva, J. J., Montoya, L., . . .Guyatt, G. H. (2018). Opioids for chronic noncancer pain: A systematic review and meta-analysis. *JAMA. 320*(23), 2448 -2460.

Centers for Disease Control and Prevention. (2017). *Opioid overdose*. Retrieved from https://www.cdc.gov/drugoverdose/opioids/prescribed.html

Centers for Disease Control and Prevention. (2018a). *CDC Guideline for prescribing opioids for chronic pain.* Retrieved from https://www.cdc.gov/drugoverdose/prescribing/guideline.html

Centers for Disease Control and Prevention. (2018b). *Opioids in the workplace: Responding to a overdose.* Retrieved from https://www.cdc.gov/niosh/topics/opioids/response.html

Centers for Disease Control and Prevention. (2019a). *CDC advises against misapplication of the guideline for prescribing opioids for chronic pain.* Retrieved from https://www.cdc.gov/media/releases/2019/s0424-advises-misapplication-guideline-prescribing-opioids.html

Centers for Disease Control and Prevention. (2019b). *Pocket guide: Tapering opioids for chronic pain.* National Institutes of Health. Atlanta, GA: Author. Retrieved from https://www.cdc.gov/drugoverdose/pdf/clinical_pocket_guide_tapering-a.pdf

Centers for Disease Control and Prevention. (2019c). *Vital signs.* Retrieved from https://www.cdc.gov/vitalsigns/naloxone/index.html

Chutuape, M. A., Jasinski, D. R., Fingerhood, M. I., & Stitzer, M. L. (2001). One-, three-, and six-month outcomes after brief inpatient opioid detoxification. *The American Journal of Drug and Alcohol Abuse, 27*(1), 19–44.

Ciccarone, D. (2017). Fentanyl in the US heroin supply: A rapidly changing risk environment. *The International Journal on Drug Policy, 46,* 107–111.

Clark, A. K., Wilder, C. M., & Winstanley, E. L. (2014). A systematic review of community opioid overdose prevention and naloxone distribution programs. *Journal of Addiction Medicine, 8*(3), 153–163.

Cohen, B. R., Mahoney, K. M., Baro, E., Squire, C., Beck, M., Travis, S., . . . Woodcock, J. (2020). FDA initiative for drug facts label for over-the-counter naloxone. *New England Journal of Medicine, 382*(22), 2129–2136.

Comer, S., Cunningham, C., Fishman, M. J., Gordon, F. A., Kampman, F. K., Langleben, D., . . . Wright, T. J. (2015). National practice guideline for the use of medications in the treatment of addiction involving opioid use. *The American Society of Addiction Medicine, 66.*

Cornish, R., Macleod, J., Strang, J., Vickerman, P., & Hickman, M. (2010). Risk of death during and after opiate substitution treatment in primary care: Prospective observational study in UK General Practice Research Database. *BMJ, 341,* c5475.

Davis, D. R., Kurti, A. N., Skelly, J. M., Redner, R., White, T. J., & Higgins, S. T. (2016). A review of the literature on contingency management in the treatment of substance use disorders. *Preventive Medicine 2009–2014. 92,* 36–46.

Davison, J. W., Sweeney, M. L., Bush, K. R., Correale, T. M., Calsyn, D. A., Reoux, J. P., . . . Kivlahan, D. R. (2006). Outpatient treatment engagement and abstinence rates following inpatient opioid detoxification. *Journal of Addictive Diseases, 25*(4), 27–35. doi:10.1300/J069v25n04_03

Devereaux, A. L., Mercer, S. L., & Cunningham, C. W. (2018). Dark classics in chemical neuroscience: morphine. *ACS Chemical Neuroscience, 9*(10), 2395–2407.

Deyo, R. A., Hallvik, S. E., Hildebran, C., Marino, M., Dexter, E., Irvine, J. M., . . . Leichtling, G. J. (2017). Association between initial opioid prescribing patterns and subsequent long-term use among opioid-naïve patients: A statewide retrospective cohort study. *Journal of General Internal Medicine, 32*(1), 21–27.

Diaper, A. M., Law, F. D., & Melichar, J. K. (2014). Pharmacological strategies for detoxification. *British Journal of Clinical Pharmacology, 77*(2), 302–314.

Dowell, D., Haegerich, T., & Chou, R. (2016). CDC guideline for prescribing opioids for chronic pain—United States, 2016. *MMWR Recommendations and Reports, 65*(No. RR-1), 1–49. doi:10.15585/mmwr.rr6501e1

Drug Enforcement Agency. (2020). DEA drug facts. Retrieved from https://www.dea.gov/factsheets?field_fact_sheet_category_target_id=331

Dugosh, K., Abraham, A., Seymour, B., McLoyd, K., Chalk, M., & Festinger, D. J. (2016). A systematic review on the use of psychosocial interventions in conjunction with medications for the treatment of opioid addiction. *Journal of Addiction Medicine, 10*(2), 91–101.

Dutra, L., Stathopoulou, G., Basden, S. L., Leyro, T. M., Powers, M. B., & Otto, M. W. (2008). A meta-analytic review of psychosocial interventions for substance use disorders. *American Journal of Psychiatry, 165*(2), 179–187. doi:10.1176/appi.ajp.2007.06111851

D'Onofrio, G., O'Connor, P. G., Pantalon, M. V., Chawarski, M. C., Busch, S. H., Owens, P. H., . . . Fiellin, D. A. (2015). Emergency department–initiated buprenorphine/naloxone treatment for opioid dependence: A randomized clinical trial. *JAMA, 313*(16), 1636–1644.

Faggiano, F., Vigna-Taglianti, F., Versino, E., & Lemma, P. J. (2003). Methadone maintenance at different dosages for opioid dependence. *Cochrane Database of Sytematic Reviews*, (3). https://doi.org/10.1002/14651858.CD002208

Ferri, M., Amato, L., & Davoli, M. J. (2006). Alcoholics Anonymous and other 12-step programmes for alcohol dependence. *Cochrane Database of Systematic Reviews*, (3). https://doi.org/10.1002/14651858.CD005032.pub2

Fiellin, D. A., Barry, D. T., Sullivan, L. E., Cutter, C. J., Moore, B. A., O'Connor, P. G., & Schottenfeld, R. S. (2013). A randomized trial of cognitive behavioral therapy in primary care-based buprenorphine. *The American Journal of Medicine*, *126*(1), 74.e11–74.e17.

Finnerup, N. B. (2019). Nonnarcotic methods of pain management. *New England Journal of Medicine, 380*(25), 2440–2448.

First, M. B. (2009). Harmonisation of ICD-11 and DSM-V: Opportunities and challenges. *British Journal of Psychiatry , 195*(5), 382–390. doi:10.1192/bjp.bp.108.060822

Fudin, J. (2018a). Opioid Agonists, Partial Agonists, Antagonists: Oh My! Retrieved from https://www.pharmacytimes.com/contributor/jeffrey-fudin/2018/01/opioid-agonists-partial-agonists-antagonists-oh-my

Furlan, A. D., Chaparro, L. E., Irvin, E., & Mailis-Gagnon, A. (2011). A comparison between enriched and nonenriched enrollment randomized withdrawal trials of opioids for chronic noncancer pain. *Journal of Pain Research and Management, 16*(5), 337–351.

Ghatak, S. (2010). "The Opium Wars": The biopolitics of narcotic control in the United States, 1914–1935. *Critical Criminology, 18*(1), 41–56.

Gowing, L., Ali, R., White, J. M., & Mbewe, D. J. (2017). Buprenorphine for managing opioid withdrawal. *Cochrane Database of Systematic Reviews*, (2).

Haley, S. J., Dugosh, K. L., & Lynch, K. G. (2011). Performance contracting to engage detoxification-only patients into continued rehabilitation. *Journal of Substance Abuse Treatment, 40*(2), 123–131.

Haley, S. J., Maroko, A. R., Wyka, K., & Baker, M. R. (2019). The association between county-level safety net treatment access and opioid hospitalizations and mortality in New York. *Journal of Substance Abuse Treatment, 100*, 52–58.

Hopper, J., Wu, J., Martus, W., & Pierre, J. (2005). A randomized trial of one-day vs. three-day buprenorphine inpatient detoxification protocols for heroin dependence. *Journal of Opioid Management, 1*(1), 31–35.

Hosztafi, S. (2001). The history of heroin. *Acta Pharmaceutica Hungarica, 71*(2), 233–242.

How Profits From Opium Shaped 19th-Century Boston - Part 1 (2017) Retrieved from https://www.wbur.org/commonhealth/2017/07/31/opium-boston-history

Hunt, G. M., Azrin, N. H. (1973). A community-reinforcement approach to alcoholism. *Behavior Reseach and Therapy, 11*(1), 91–104.

Hutchinson, E., Catlin, M., Andrilla, C. H. A., Baldwin, L.M., & Rosenblatt, R. A. (2014). Barriers to primary care physicians prescribing buprenorphine. *Annals of Family Medicine, 12*(2), 128–133.

Institute of Medicine. (1988). *The future of public health*. Washington, DC: The National Academies Press. doi:10.17226/1091

International Association for the Study of Pain. (1986). Classification of chronic pain. Descriptions of chronic pain syndromes and definitions of pain terms. *Pain, Suppl 3*, S1–226.

Jones, C. M., Campopiano, M., Baldwin, G., & McCance-Katz, E. (2015). National and state treatment need and capacity for opioid agonist medication-assisted treatment. *American journal of public health, 105*(8), e55–e63.

Kerensky, T., & Walley, A. Y. (2017). Opioid overdose prevention and naloxone rescue kits: What we know and what we don't know. *Addiction Science & Clinical Practice, 12*(1), 4.

Kindig, D., & Stoddart, G. J. (2003). What is population health? *American Journal of Public Health, 93*(3), 380–383. doi:10.2105/AJPH.93.3.380

Kleber, H. D. (2007). Pharmacologic treatments for opioid dependence: Detoxification and maintenance options. *Dialogues in Clinical Neuroscience, 9*(4), 455–470. Retrieved from https://www.ncbi.nlm.nih.gov/pubmed/18286804; https://www.ncbi.nlm.nih.gov/pmc/articles/PMC3202507/

Kleber, H., D. & Riordan, C. J. (1982). The treatment of narcotic withdrawal: A historical review. *The Journal of Clinical Psychiatry, 43*(6 Pt 2), 30–34.

Knudsen, H. K., & Roman, P. M. (2012). Financial factors and the implementation of medications for treating opioid use disorders. *Journal of Addiction Medicine, 6*(4), 280.

Knudsen, H. K., Havens, J. R., Lofwall, M. R., Studts, J. L., Walsh, S. L. (2017). Buprenorphine physician supply: Relationship with state-level prescription opioid mortality. *Drug and Alcohol Dependence, 173,* S55–S64.

Knudsen, H. K., Roman, P. M., & Oser, C. B. (2010). Facilitating factors and barriers to the use of medications in publicly funded addiction treatment organizations. *Journal of Addiction Medicine, 4*(2), 99.

Kosten, T. R., & George, T. P. (2002). The neurobiology of opioid dependence: Implications for treatment. *Science &Practice Perspectives, 1*(1), 13–20. Retrieved from https://www.ncbi.nlm.nih.gov/pubmed/18567959; https://www.ncbi.nlm.nih.gov/pmc/articles/PMC2851054/

Ling, W., Amass, L., Shoptaw, S., Annon, J. J., Hillhouse, M., Babcock, D., . . . Muir, J. (2005). A multi-center randomized trial of buprenorphine–naloxone versus clonidine for opioid, detoxification: Findings from the National Institute on Drug Abuse Clinical Trials Network. *Addiction, 100*(8), 1090–1100.

Macy, B. (2018). *Dopesick: Dealers, doctors, and the drug company that addicted America.* Little, Brown: Boston, MA.

Madras, B. K., Ahmad, N. J., Wen, J., & Sharfstein, J. (2020). Improving access to evidence-based medical treatment for opioid use disorder: Strategies to address key barriers within the treatment system. *National Academy of Medicine Perspectives.*

Mancher, M., & Leshner, A. (Eds.). (2019). *Medications for opioid use disorder save lives.* Washington, DC: National Academies Press. doi:10.17226/25310

Mark, T., Dilonardo, J., Chalk, M., & Coffey, R. (2002). Substance abuse detoxification: Improvements needed in linkage to treatment. Rockville, MD: Center for Substance Abuse Treatment Substance Abuse and Mental Health Services Administration.

Mark, T. L., Yee, T., Levit, K. R., Camacho-Cook, J., Cutler, E., & Carroll, C. D. (2016). Insurance financing increased for mental health conditions but not for substance use disorders, 1986–2014. *Health Affairs, 35*(6), 958–965.

Martin, S. A., Chiodo, L. M., Bosse, J. D., & Wilson, A. (2018). The next stage of buprenorphine care for opioid use disorder. *Annals of Internal Medicine, 169*(9), 628–635. doi:10.7326/m18-1652

Mattick, R. P., & Hall, W. (1996). Are detoxification programmes effective? *Lancet, 347*(8994), 97–100. doi:10.1016/s0140-6736(96)90215-9

Mattick, R. P., Breen, C., Kimber, J., & Davoli, M. (2014). Buprenorphine maintenance versus placebo or methadone maintenance for opioid dependence. *Cochrane Database of Systematic Reviews,* (2).

Mattick, R. P., Breen, C., Kimber, J., & Davoli, M. J. (2009). Methadone maintenance therapy versus no opioid replacement therapy for opioid dependence. *Cochrane Database of Systematic Reviews,* (3).

McDonald, R., & Strang, J. (2016). Are take-home naloxone programmes effective? Systematic review utilizing application of the Bradford Hill criteria. *Addiction, 111*(7), 1177–1187.

McLellan, A. T., Arndt, I. O., Metzger, D. S., Woody, G. E., & O'Brien, C. P. (1993). The effects of psychosocial services in substance abuse treatment. *Addictions Nursing Network, 5*(2), 38–47.

McLellan, A. T., Lewis, D. C., O'Brien , C. P., & Kleber, H. D. (2000). Drug dependence, a chronic medical illness: Implications for treatment, insurance, and outcomes evaluation. *JAMA, 284*(13), 1689–1695.

McLellan, A. T., & Meyers, K. (2004). Contemporary addiction treatment: A review of systems problems for adults and adolescents. *Biological Psychiatry, 56*(10), 764–770.

Medicaid Innovation Accelerator Program. (2017). Overview of substance use disorder (SUD) care clinical guidelines: A resource for states developing SUD delivery system reforms. Rockville, MD: American Society of Addiction Medicine. Retrieved from https://www.medicaid.gov/state-resource-center/innovation-accelerator-program/iap-downloads/reducing-substance-use-disorders/asam-resource-guide.pdf

Mee-Lee, D. (2013). *The ASAM criteria.* Chevy Chase, MD: American Society of Addiction Medicine.

Meyers, R. J., Roozen, H. G., Smith, J. E.. (2011). *The community reinforcement approach: An update of the evidence. Alcohol, Research & Health, 33*(4), 380.

Minozzi, S., Amato, L., Vecchi, S., Davoli, M., Kirchmayer, U., & Verster, A. J. (2011). Oral naltrexone maintenance treatment for opioid dependence. *Cochrane Database of Systematic Reviews,* (4).

Moore, B. A., Fiellin, D. A., Cutter, C. J., Buono, F. D., Barry, D. T., Fiellin, L. E., . . . Schottenfeld, R. S. (2016). Cognitive behavioral therapy improves treatment outcomes for prescription opioid users in primary care buprenorphine treatment. *Journal of Substance Abuse Treatment, 71,* 54–57.

Murphy, S., & Irwin, J. (1992). "Living with the dirty secret": Problems of disclosure for methadone maintenance clients. *Journal of Psychoactive Drugs, 24*(3), 257–264.

Musto, D. F. (1999). *The American disease: Origins of narcotic control.* New York, NY: Oxford University Press.

National Institute on Drug Abuse. (2017). Naloxone for opioid overdose: Life-saving science. Retrieved from https://www.drugabuse.gov/publications/naloxone-opioid-overdose-life-saving -science

National Institute on Drug Abuse. (2018a). *Principles of Drug Addiction Treatment: A Research-Based Guide (Third Edition).* Rockville, MD: Department of Health and Human Services. Retrieved from https://www.drugabuse.gov/download/675/principles-drug-addiction-treatment-research -based-guide-third-edition.pdf?v=87ecd1341039d24b0fd616c5589c2095

National Institute on Drug Abuse. (2018b). *Principles of Drug Addiction Treatment: A Research-Based Guide.* Rockville, MD: National Institutes of Health. Retrieved from https://www.drugabuse .gov/node/pdf/675/principles-of-drug-addiction-treatment-a-research-based-guide-third -edition

National Institute on Drug Abuse. (2018c). The science of drug use and addiction: The basics. *Media Guide.* Retrieved from https://www.drugabuse.gov/publications/media-guide/science-drug-use -addiction-basics

National Institute on Drug Abuse. (2019). The neurobiology of drug addiction. Retrieved from https://www.drugabuse.gov/publications/teaching-packets/neurobiology-drug-addiction /section-iii-action-heroin-morphine/10-addiction-vs-dependence

National Institutes of Health. (2019). The role of opioids in the treatment of chronic pain. *Pathways to Prevention (P2P): Workshop Program.* Retrieved from https://prevention.nih.gov/research -priorities/research-needs-and-gaps/pathways-prevention/role-opioids-treatment-chronic -pain

Norn, S., Kruse, P. R., & Kruse, E. (2005). History of opium poppy and morphine. *Dan Medicinhist Arbog, 33,* 171–184.

O'Connor, P. G. (2005). Methods of detoxification and their role in treating patients with opioid dependence. *JAMA, 294*(8), 961–963.

Oelhaf, R. C., Azadfard, M., & Kum, B. (2019). Opioid toxicity. In *StatPearls [Internet]:* StatPearls Publishing. Retrieved from https://www.ncbi.nlm.nih.gov/books/NBK431077/

Office of The Assistant Secretary for Planning and Evaluation. (2019). *Psychosocial Supports in Medication-Assisted Treatment: Recent Evidence and Current Practice.* Retrieved from https:// aspe.hhs.gov/basic-report/psychosocial-supports-medication-assisted-treatment-recent -evidence-and-current-practice

Petersen, A., & Lupton, D. (1996). *The New Public Health : Health and Self in the Age of Risk:* SAGE.

Petry, N. M. (2000). A comprehensive guide to the application of contingency management procedures in clinical settings. *Drug and Alcohol Dependence, 58*(1–2), 9–25.

Pleuvry, B. J. (2004). Receptors, agonists and antagonists. *Anaesthesia & Intensive Care Medicine, 5*(10), 350–352.

Poon, L. (2017). Opium dens are a terrible theme for bars. *City Lab.* Retrieved from https://www .citylab.com/life/2017/05/the-opium-dens-of-chinatown/528108

Redford, A., & Powell, B. (2016). Dynamics of intervention in the war on drugs: The buildup to the Harrison Act of 1914. *The Independent Review, 20*(4), 509–530.

Rees, D. I., Sabia, J. J., Argys, L. M., Latshaw, J., & Dave, D. (2017). *With a little help from my friends: The effects of Naloxone access and Good Samaritan laws on opioid-related deaths.* Retrieved from https://www.nber.org/papers/w23171

Rivat, C., & Ballantyne, J. (2016). The dark side of opioids in pain management: Basic science explains clinical observation. *Pain Reports, 1*(2), e570. doi:10.1097/PR9.0000000000000570

Robins, L., Helzer, J., Hesselbrock, M., & Wish, E. (2010). Vietnam veterans three years after Vietnam: How our study changed our view of heroin. *The American Journal on Addictions, 19*(3), 203.

Satel, S. L., Kosten, T. R., Schuckit, M. A., & Fischman, M. W. (1993). Should protracted withdrawal from drugs be included in DSM-IV? *The American Journal of Psychiatry, 150*(5), 695–704. doi:10.1176/ajp.150.5.695

Saunders, J. B. (2017). Substance use and addictive disorders in DSM-5 and ICD 10 and the draft ICD 11. *Current Opinion in Psychiatry, 30*(4), 227–237. doi:10.1097/yco.0000000000000332

Schuckit, M. A. (2016). Treatment of opioid-use disorders. *New England Journal of Medicine, 375*(4), 357–368.

Shah, A. H., Corey, J., Martin, B. C. (2017). *Characteristics of initial prescription episodes and likelihood of long-term opioid use — United States, 2006–2015.* Retrieved from https://www.cdc .gov/mmwr/volumes/66/wr/mm6610a1.htm#F1_down

Sigmon, S. C., Bisaga, A., Nunes, E. V., O'Connor, P. G., Kosten, T., & Woody, G. (2012). Opioid detoxification and naltrexone induction strategies: Recommendations for clinical practice. *The American Journal of Drug and Alcohol Abuse, 38*(3), 187–199. doi:10.3109/00952990.2011 .653426

Sinha, R. (2001). How does stress increase risk of drug abuse and relapse? *Psychopharmacology, 158*(4), 343–359.

Sinha, R. (2008). Chronic stress, drug use, and vulnerability to addiction. *Annals of the New York Academy of Sciences, 1141*, 105.

Smyth, B. P., Barry, J., Keenan, E., & Ducray, K. (2010). Lapse and relapse following inpatient treatment of opiate dependence. *Irish Medical Journal, 103*(6), 176–179.

Stein, M. D., & Friedmann, P. D. (2007). Optimizing opioid detoxification: Rearranging deck chairs on the Titanic. *Journal of Addictive Diseases, 26*(2), 1–2. doi:10.1300/J069v26n02_01

Stobbe, M. (2017, October 28). Today's opioid crisis shares chilling similarities with past drug epidemics. *The Chicago Tribune.* Retrieved from https://www.chicagotribune.com/nation-world /ct-drug-epidemics-history-20171028-story.html

Strang, J., McCambridge, J., Best, D., Beswick, T., Bearn, J., Rees, S., & Gossop, M. (2003). Loss of tolerance and overdose mortality after inpatient opiate detoxification: Follow up study. *BMJ, 326*(7396), 959–960.

Substance Abuse and Mental Health Services Administration. (2015). *Federal guidelines for opioid treatment programs.* Rockville, MD: U.S. Department of Health and Human Services. Retrieved from https://store.samhsa.gov/sites/default/files/d7/priv/pep15-fedguideotp.pdf

Substance Abuse and Mental Health Services Administration. (2018). *Key substance use and mental health indicators in the United States: Results from the 2017 National Survey on Drug Use and Health* (HHS Publication No. SMA 18-5068, NSDUH Series H-53). Rockville, MD: Center for Behavioral Health Statistics and Quality, Substance Abuse and Mental Health Services Administration.

Substance Abuse and Mental Health Services Administration. (2019a). Apply for a practitioner waiver. Retrieved from https://www.samhsa.gov/medication-assisted-treatment/training -materials-resources/apply-for-practitioner-waiver

Substance Abuse and Mental Health Services Administration. (2019b). *Key substance use and mental health indicators in the United States: Results from the 2018 National Survey on Drug Use and Health* (HHS Publication No. PEP19-5068, NSDUH Series H-54). Rockville, MD: Center for Behavioral Health Statistics and Quality. Retrieved from https://www.samhsa .gov/data/sites/default/files/cbhsq-reports/NSDUHNationalFindingsReport2018/NSDUH NationalFindingsReport2018.pdf

Substance Abuse and Mental Health Services Administration. (2019c). *Understanding the Final Rule for a Patient Limit of 275.* Retrieved from https://www.samhsa.gov/sites/default/files /programs_campaigns/medication_assisted/understanding-patient-limit275.pdf

Substance Abuse and Mental Health Services Administration. (2020). *Opioid Treatment Program (OTP) Guidance.* Rockville, MD: Author. Retrieved from https://www.samhsa.gov/sites/default /files/otp-guidance-20200316.pdf

Tanum, L., Solli, K. K., Latif, Z.-e.-H., Benth, J. Š., Opheim, A., Sharma-Haase, K., . . . Kunøe, N. (2017). Effectiveness of injectable extended-release naltrexone vs daily buprenorphine-naloxone for opioid dependence: A randomized clinical noninferiority trial. *JAMA Psychiatry, 74*(12), 1197–1205. doi:10.1001/jamapsychiatry.2017.3206

Tempalski, B., Cleland, C. M., Williams, L. D., Cooper, H. L. F., & Friedman, S. R. (2018). Change and variability in drug treatment coverage among people who inject drugs in 90 large metropolitan areas in the USA, 1993–2007. *Substance Abuse Treatment Prevention and Policy, 13*, 7. doi:10.1186/s13011-018-0165-2

Terry, C. (1915). The Harrison anti-narcotic act. *American Journal of Public Health, 5*(6), 518. doi:10.2105/ajph.5.6.518

Tighe, T. J., & Elliott, R. (1968). A technique for controlling behavior in natural life settings. *Journal of Applied Behavior Analysis, 1*(3), 263–266.

Timko, C., Below, M., Vittorio, L., Taylor, E., Chang, G., Lash, S., . . . Brief, D. (2019). Randomized controlled trial of enhanced telephone monitoring with detoxification patients: 3- and 6-month outcomes. *Journal of Substance Abuse Treatment, 99*, 24–31. doi:10.1016/j.jsat.2018.12.008

Timko, C., Schultz, N. R., Cucciare, M. A., Vittorio, L., & Garrison-Diehn, C. (2016). Retention in medication-assisted treatment for opiate dependence: A systematic review. *Journal of Addictive Diseases, 35*(1), 22–35. doi:10.1080/10550887.2016.1100960

Trafton, J. A., Minkel, J., & Humphreys, K. (2006). Determining effective methadone doses for individual opioid-dependent patients. PLoS *Medicine, 3*(3), e80. doi:10.1371/journal.pmed .0030080

Turnock, B. (2011). *Essentials of public health.* Burlington, MA: Jones & Bartlett Publishers.

U.S. Department of Health and Human Services, Office of the Secretary. (2021). *Practice Guidelines for the Administration of Buprenorphine for Treating Opioid Use Disorder.* Retrieved from: HYPERLINK "https://urldefense.proofpoint.com/v2/url?u=https-3A__www.hhs.gov_sites _default_files_mat-2Dphysician-2Dpractice-2Dguidelines.pdf&d=DwMFAg&c=mRWFL96 tuqj9V0Jjj4h40ddo0XsmttALwKjAEOCyUjY&r=w8kfi6iGAuKmSdBQX1tROVjXWu2AM3q EW73g-3A353I&m=DUVDguGw7LhD_WhRf_BsEdQTcrrnat5W9TR8sz4I1b4&s=iRKL6Mq KTOKBjqFRL8VoewmpCLFCBu95CYz59dWY0fI&e=" https://www.hhs.gov/sites/default/files /mat-physician-practice-guidelines.pdf

U.S. Food and Drug Administration. (2018). *FDA identifies harm reported from sudden discontinuation of opioid pain medicines and requires label changes to guide prescribers on gradual, individualized tapering.* Retrieved from https://www.fda.gov/drugs/drug-safety-and -availability/fda-identifies-harm-reported-sudden-discontinuation-opioid-pain-medicines -and-requires-label-changes

U.S. Food and Drug Administration. (2018). *Joint Meeting of the Anesthetic and Analgesic Drug Products Advisory Committee and the Drug Safety and Risk Management Advisory Committee.* Silver Spring, MD. Retrieved from https://www.fda.gov/advisory-committees/anesthetic -and-analgesic-drug-products-advisory-committee/2018-meeting-materials-anesthetic-and -analgesic-drug-products-advisory-committee

U.S. Food and Drug Administration. (2019). FDA identifies harm reported from sudden discontinuation of opioid pain medicines and requires label changes to guide prescribers on gradual, individualized tapering. Retrieved from https://www.fda.gov/drugs/drug-safety-and -availability/fda-identifies-harm-reported-sudden-discontinuation-opioid-pain-medicines-and -requires-label-changes

U.S. Food and Drug Administration. (2019). Part I: The 1906 Food and Drugs Act and Its Enforcement. Retrieved from https://www.fda.gov/about-fda/fdas-evolving-regulatory-powers /part-i-1906-food-and-drugs-act-and-its-enforcement

U.S. Food and Drug Administration. (2020a). About FDA. Retrieved from https://www.fda.gov /about-fda

U.S. Food and Drug Administration. (2020b). Center for Drug Evaluation and Research. Retrieved from https://www.fda.gov/about-fda/fda-organization/center-drug-evaluation-and-research-cder

Wein, H. (Ed.). (2015). Biology of addiction. *NIH News in Health.* Retrieved from https:// newsinhealth.nih.gov/sites/nihNIH/files/2015/October/NIHNiHOct2015.pdf

World Health Organization. (1993). *The ICD-10 classification of mental and behavioural disorders: Diagnostic criteria for research* (Vol. 2): Geneva, Switzerland: World Health Organization.

World Health Organization. (2009a). *Clinical guidelines for withdrawal management and treatment of drug dependence in closed settings.* Geneva, Switzerland: World Health Organization.

World Health Organization. (2009b). *Guidelines for the psychosocially assisted pharmacological treatment of opioid dependence.* Geneva, Switzerland: World Health Organization.

World Health Organization. (2013). *Opioid overdose: Preventing and reducing opioid overdose mortality*. Geneva, Switzerland: World Health Organization. Retrieved from https://www.unodc.org /docs/treatment/overdose.pdf

World Health Organization. (2017). Community management of opioid overdose 2014. Retrieved from http://apps.who.int/iris/bitstream/10665/137462/1/9789241548816_eng. pdf

World Health Organization. (2018). *International classification of diseases for mortality and morbidity statistics (11th Revision)*. Geneva, Switzerland: World Health Organization. Retrieved from https://icd.who.int/en

Zhang, Z., Friedmann, P. D., & Gerstein, D. R. (2003). Does retention matter? Treatment duration and improvement in drug use. *Addiction, 98*(5), 673–684. doi:10.1046/j.1360-0443.2003.00354.x

CHAPTER 2

How Did We Get Here?

KEY TERMS

Acute Pain
Affordable Care Act (ACA)
Analgesics
Centers for Disease Control and
  Prevention (CDC)
Clinical Trial
Controlled Substances Act (CSA)
Drug Diversion
Drug Misuse
Epidemic
Evidence-based Treatment
Harm Reduction
Iatrogenic
Indian Health Service (IHS)
Medicaid

Methadone Maintenance Treatment
  (MMT)
Morphine Milligram Equivalent (MME)
Mortality Rate
National Institute on Drug Abuse (NIDA)
Opioid Dependence
Opioid Tolerance
Prescription Drug Monitoring Programs
  (PDMP)
The Joint Commission (TJC)
U.S. Preventive Services Task Force
  (USPSTF)
Veterans Health Administration
World Health Organization (WHO)

LEARNING OBJECTIVES

- Identify the three waves of the opioid epidemic suggested by the CDC
- Describe what the authors of this text mean by suggesting that the CDC's three
  waves misses the political determinants of health
- Discuss President Nixon's role in the "War on Drugs"
- Define iatrogenic illnesses
- Explain the role of the pharmaceutical industry in the opioid epidemic
- Identify how the elevation of pain management as a medical priority is linked to
  the epidemic
- Describe various state-level interventions to curb the epidemic as well as their
  effectiveness
- Explain how the opioid epidemic impacts various healthcare delivery services and
  the associated costs

Chapter 2 reviews how the United States found its way into an opioid epidemic in the late 21st century after having experienced other opioid challenges in the 19th and 20th centuries.

Across two decades (1999–2018), nearly 450,000 people died from an opioid-related overdose. These deaths include those attributable to pharmaceutical opioids taken with and without a prescription as well as other non-prescription opioids (National Center for Health Statistics, 2020). The CDC attributes this rise in opioid overdose deaths to three distinct waves (CDC, 2020):

1. The first wave began with increased prescribing of opioids in the 1990s, with overdose deaths increasing since at least 1999.
2. The second wave began in 2010, with rapid increases in heroin overdose deaths.
3. The third wave began in 2013, with significant increases in overdose deaths involving synthetic opioids, particularly those involving fentanyl.

If one begins in 1999 and attributes overdose mortality only to differences in opioid compounds, the CDC's framing of the epidemic has merit. Please see **Figure 2-1**. However, what the CDC's "three distinct waves" framework misses is the social, economic, historical, and political context that fostered the current epidemic. Although the CDC focuses on the last two decades, opioid use, dependence, and overdose mortality have been a part of American life for centuries. America's

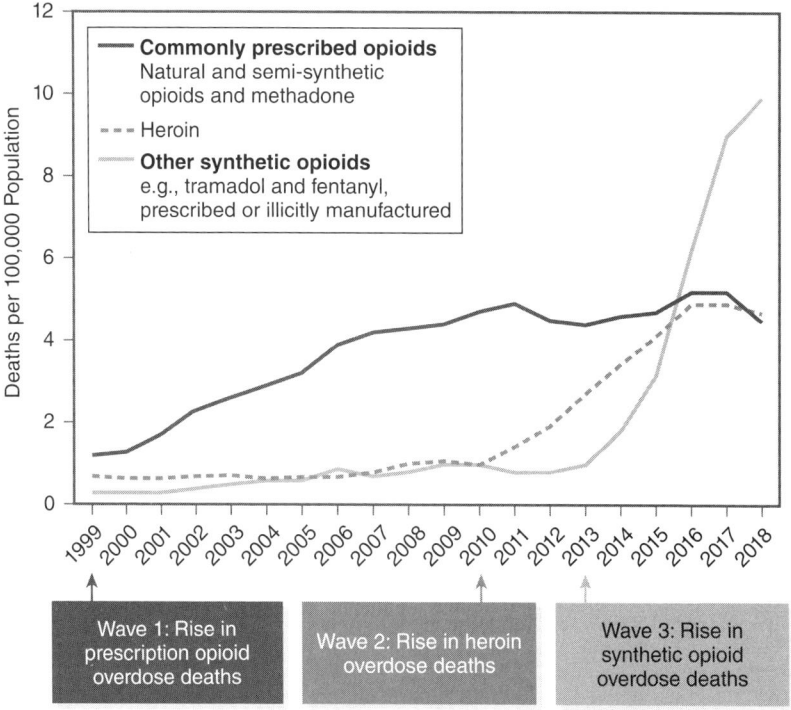

Figure 2-1 Three Waves of the Rise in Opioid Overdose Deaths.

Centers for Disease Control and Prevention. Retrieved from https://www.cdc.gov/drugoverdose/images/epidemic/2018-3-Wave-Lines-Mortality.png

history with opium and other opioids is replete with issues of who controls their production, marketing, and profits, as well as the disparate impact associated with gender, race, and class. It is important to circle back to a time before 1999 to illustrate how the current epidemic holds echoes from our past and transcends the CDC's three waves.

An 1833 letter to the editor in *The Boston Medical and Surgical Journal* (which became the *New England Journal of Medicine*) solicited readership for help in treating opioid addiction (Seeger, 1833). The letter stated that the patient initiated opioid use specifically for medical reasons, and not for "unnatural excitement of inebriation," and that opioid use continued out of necessity, i.e., a state of dependence. The article triggered an outpouring of responses from physicians whose patients were struggling with similar issues. They wrote of patients who had initiated opium use and become dependent either through physicians' orders, those who aquired an opiate directly through a pharmacist (Bebinger, 2017b).

> "When we allude to opium eaters, we mean those only who took it originally as a medicine for some nervous affection, and continue it from necessity, rather than from choice;—who take it, not to intoxicate, but to strengthen and balance the nervous system and enable them to attend to business, and to appear like other people. Of those who take opium for purposes of unnatural excitement and inebriation, we have no knowledge."
>
> **"Opium Eating"** (1833)

It is important to remember that at the time, physicians and pharmacists did not have many medications and opium was among the most popular treatments. It was often dispensed in tablet or liquid form, the latter known as laudanum, to treat headaches, insomnia, diarrhea, stomach pains, cholera, or a toothache. Please see **Figure 2-2**. Although generous profits were certainly made on domestic retail sales, American merchants also made an abundance of money from the opium trade in the middle of the 19th century.

Although both Opium Wars (1839–1860) were fought between the British and Chinese Governments over Britain's imposition of the opium trade on China, Americans controlled approximately 10% of the trade. Turkish opium was brought to China for sale, and American ships returned to the United States with Chinese goods such as silk and opium. In just one year, one Boston trading company made the equivalent of 25 million U.S. dollars on opium sales. The opium trade became a central source of wealth for several of America's richest East Coast families including the Cabots, Cushings, Welds, Delanos (the grandfather of President Franklin Delano Roosevelt), and Forbes (Bebinger, 2017a). Although opium use in the United States would increase through the middle of the 19th century, it was not until the Civil War (1861–1865) when morphine was widely distributed to wounded Confederate and Union soldiers that a second opioid surge took hold.

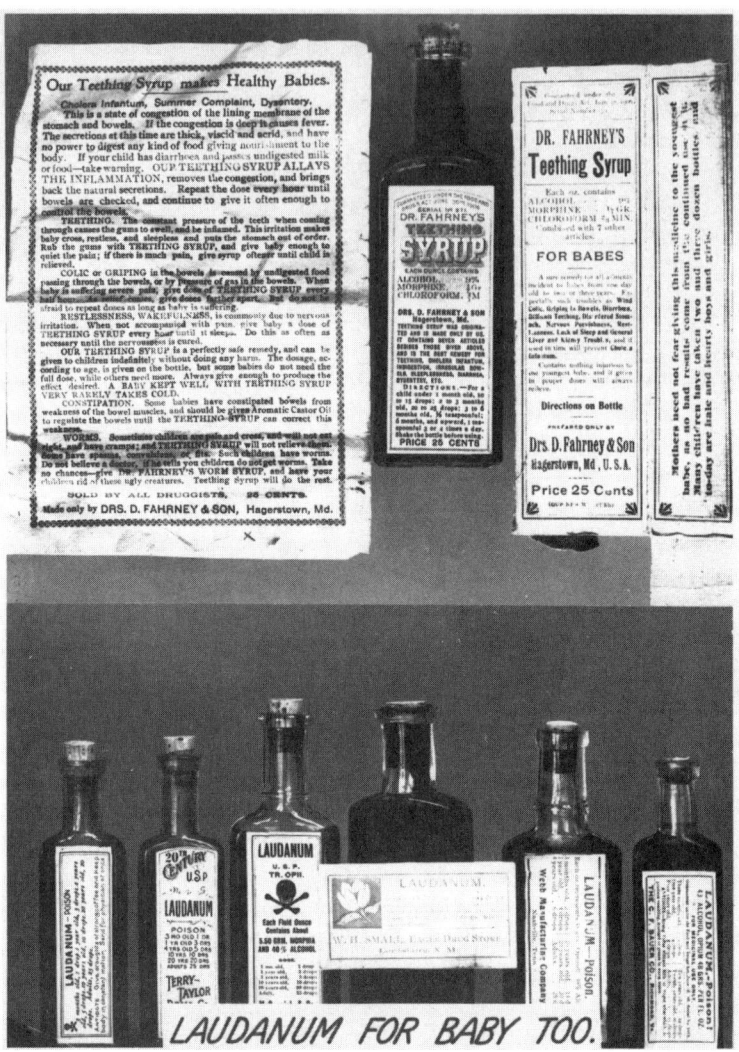

Figure 2-2 Display of Various Patent Medicines for Teething Babies.

It would be several decades after the end of the Civil War that federal law would begin to address opioid revenues to curb availability and use. The 1914 Harrison Act focused on taxation but not the outright prohibition of opium. The imposition of higher taxes increased prices and discouraged consumption, which reduced supply. According to some historians, the epidemic of the late 19th century had started a downward turn before the Harrison Act passed as physicians and pharmacists became less generous in making the drug available (Tricker, 2018). With less availability and no ready substitute, the epidemic began to subside (Bebinger, 2017b). By the 1930s and 1940s, heroin use had further abated as the Great Depression and World War II interfered with demand and supply chains, forcing some to turn to pharmaceuticals (morphine and methadone) (Hughes, Barker, Crawford, & Jaffe, 1972).

Although there is evidence that heroin use started to increase again between the end of WWII and the start of the Vietnam War, the escalation quickened in the later years of the Vietnam War. Estimates suggest that almost half of those deployed in Vietnam tried heroin at least once and that just under half of those became dependent (Robins, 1974). The National Institute on Drug Abuse estimates that from 1969 to 1974, the number of heroin addicts in the United States more than doubled, rising from 242,000 to 558,000. By the mid-1970s the New York City Health Department was reporting more than 650 heroin-related deaths a year (Kerr, 1986).

Political Determinants and the Opioid Epidemic

Although the most recent opioid epidemic is often discussed as "the opioid epidemic," such framing obscures the country's long relationship with opioids. As discussed in Chapter 1, the country's opioid history is strongly connected to polictical decisions, and those decisions are associated with specific opioid compounds (pharmaceutical opioids and heroin), and the compounds have long been linked by politicians, industry, and the media to race and class identities (Netherland & Hansen, 2016). For example, from 1979 to 2015, the opioid mortality rate for Whites increased from 0.44 to 12 per 100,000 representing an average increase of 10% per year, while the rate for Blacks increased from 0.62 to 6.6 for an average annual increase of 6%. Although the rate for Whites increased continuously, the rate for Blacks remained stable from 1994 until 2011 at about the time when fentanyl became more available (Alexander, Kiang, & Barbieri, 2018). Why was there such a dramatic increase over a relatively short time span and why were there such pronounced differences by race?

Racial disparities in opioid-related mortality are not new. What has changed is that over the last 40 years rapid changes in the availability and marketing of pharmaceutical opioids created demand that remained even when availability was curtailed and prices increased. For example, the mortality rate from opioids other than heroin (pharmaceutical opioids) increased in the period between 1979 to 2015 from approximately 0.25 for Whites and Blacks to 8.2 for Whites and 4.2 for Blacks. The rate increased substantially from 1993–2010 for Whites but remained stable for Blacks. However, during 2013–2015, mortality spiked for both populations, at an annual rate of 18% for Whites and 34% for Blacks (Alexander et al., 2018).

Opioid mortality rates did not just differ for pharmaceutical opioids, rates also differed for heroin. In 1979, the heroin mortality rate was 0.14 for Whites and 0.33 for Blacks (per 100,000); African Americans were dying from heroin at more than double the White rate. By 2015, Whites had higher rates: the heroin mortality rates had risen to 4.8 for Whites and 3.1 for Blacks, representing average annual increases of 12% for Whites and 7% for Blacks (Alexander et al., 2018). Between 2010 and 2015, the annual percent change in heroin mortality crossed over 30% for both Black and White populations (Alexander et al., 2018). It is worth noting that in 2017, the United States Council of Economic Advisors estimated that by 2015, the economic cost of the opioid crisis was $504 billion, or nearly 3% percent of the Gross Domestic Product (Council of Economic Advisors, 2017).

What was happening to contribute to these mortality trends? If one looks further back in the timeline from the one offered by the CDC, one can explore how opioid use was characterized, and how those characterizations relate to overdose deaths.

Beginning in 1979, the opioid epidemic can be divided into an alternative set of three waves. During the first wave, from 1979 to the mid-1990s, opioid mortality was higher for African Americans and rates of increase were nearly similar for Whites and African Americans, largely driven by heroin. From the mid-1990s to 2010, the second wave, the prescription painkiller epidemic expanded quickly among Whites while opioid mortality remained largely stable among African Americans. As a result, by 2010 the opioid mortality rate was more than two times higher for Whites than for Blacks—a reversal from just a few years earlier. In the latest wave, from about 2010 to 2017, the opioid mortality rate grew rapidly for both the Black and White populations nationally, driven by pharmaceuticals and then heroin, and more recently by synthetic opioids (Alexander et al., 2018). For those interested, a similar historic trend has been identified in NYC (Allen, Nolan, Kunins, & Paone, 2019).

Part 1: The "War on Drugs," "Street Crime," and Racial Tropes

There are many contributing factors to the opioid epidemic(s), but a core feature involves the characterization of drugs and race. One such characterization involved a calculated political strategy in 1969 that used heroin as a vehicle to undercut African American communities. In a special address to Congress in July 1969, President Richard Nixon launched the United States' War on Drugs, not as a comprehensive prevention and treatment initiative, but as a criminal justice priority (Nixon, 1969). The Nixon quotation below is illustrative of how heroin was used to link drugs, crime, and urban centers. The term "street crime" was coded language used to mean urban neighborhoods populated by people of color.

> "The habit of the narcotics addict is not only a danger to himself, but a threat to the community where he lives. Narcotics have been cited as a primary cause of the enormous increase in street crimes over the last decade.
>
> As the addict's tolerance for drugs increases, his demand for drugs rises, and the cost of his habit grows. It can easily reach hundreds of dollars a day. Since an underworld "fence" will give him only a fraction of the value of goods he steals, an addict can be forced to commit two or three burglaries a day to maintain his habit. Street robberies, prostitution, even the enticing of others into addiction to drugs—an addict will reduce himself to any offense, any degradation in order to acquire the drugs he craves."
>
> **Nixon, R.** (1969)

In the decades that followed, lawmakers at every level of government promoted harsher sentencing laws and increased enforcement actions including those targeting low-level drug offenses (Whitford & Yates, 2009). The enforcement systems that maintained these policies often focused on poor neighborhoods where public interactions and transactions were more visible. In 1994, decades after the "War on Drugs'" was announced and the criminal justice system expanded, a key Nixon presidential advisor, John Ehrlichman, admitted that Nixon's "War on Drugs" was a political strategy to destabilize specific communities, including African Americans. Please see the Ehrlichman quotation below.

> *"The Nixon campaign in 1968, and the Nixon White House after that, had two enemies: the antiwar left and black people. You understand what I'm saying? We knew we couldn't make it illegal to be either against the war or black, but by getting the public to associate the hippies with marijuana and blacks with heroin, and then criminalizing both heavily, we could disrupt those communities. We could arrest their leaders, raid their homes, break up their meetings, and vilify them night after night on the evening news. Did we know we were lying about the drugs? Of course we did."*
>
> **John Ehrlichman**, Richard Nixon's Domestic Policy Advisor
> (as cited in Baum, 1994)

Heroin is Not a Domestic Product

As with 19th century opium, the United States continued to import opioids (in the form of heroin) in later centuries—it is not grown in the United States. As demand in the United States increased, heroin siezures increased by 87% between 2009 and 2013 (Drug Enforcement Administation, 2015).

At issue here is not the origin, but heroin's availability. Since 2010, greater availability of heroin has been accompanied by an increase in purity and a decline in price (Office of National Drug Control Policy, 2015). Like other products, the availability (supply) of heroin is related to price and use. When there is an abundance of heroin, the price drops, which can encourage individuals to switch to it when the availability of a different but familiar opioid, such as a prescription opioid, contracts (which happens when insurance companies reduce their willingness to pay for it or prescribers become less willing to prescribe). The contraction in the availability of prescription opioids increases demand for that opioid, and as demand goes up, the price follows. Alternatively, the greater the availability (supply) of heroin, the lower the cost.

As suggested by the CDC, heroin's availability and low cost have been consequential. For example, in NYC, which historically has had higher rates of heroin use (Kerr, 1986), there were 1,444 drug overdose deaths in 2018—the first time in seven consecutive years that there had been a drop in opioid-related mortality. Eighty percent of those deaths in 2018 involved an opioid (1,155) and about half (51%) of those deaths involved heroin. By those calculations, 589 people died of a heroin-related death in NYC in 2018 with a population of about 8.4 million. By comparison, in the mid-1970s when the city had nearly the same population (7.9 million), the number of heroin related deaths was 650 (Kerr, 1986). Again, heroin is not a domestic product and it was readily available 50 years ago. The CDC's three-wave framing of the opioid epidemic that begins in the 1990s may obscure earlier signals of population level harms.

Increases in heroin availability, purity, and reductions in price have been temporally associated with the increases in heroin use and dependence, as well as mortality (Jones, Logan, Gladden, & Bohm, 2015). As described in the next section, increases in heroin availability, purity, and reductions in price coincided with the relatively, recent period when medicine was experiencing growing pressure to reduce the seemingly limitless supply of opioid prescriptions.

Part 2: Big Pharma, Pain, and Poor People

Iatrogenic illnesses are those illnesses caused by medical examination or treatment. This definition is important because the second explanation for increases in opioid-related mortality has to do with the how history (and science) seemed to forget about the addictive properties of opioids, and the role that profit motives play in creating demand. The second portion of the epidemic is related to the iatrogenic effects of the widespread use of pharmaceutical opioids to treat non-cancer related pain.

Pain is a considerable health problem. An estimated 25 million adult Americans suffer daily from pain and 23 million others suffer from severe recurrent pain (Meldrum, 2016). Pain management is a vast topic, and a detailed description of its appropriate medical management is beyond the scope of this work. The following is a brief overview.

A multidisciplinary team approach involving physical and psychological therapies, including cognitive-behavioral therapy, relaxation, pain coping skills training, and self-hypnosis are the best-known alternative to opioids. However, insurance companies rarely cover the costs of such a comprehensive treatment approach. When they do, financial coverage is often insufficient, and many communities do not have the resources to support a multi-disciplinary approach if they do not have a major medical center (Meldrum, 2016). Within that context, it is important to provide a brief overview of how prescription pain medications proliferated. In short, several pharmaceutical companies promoted opioid pain medication, targeted the working poor and discounted associated risks, as government agencies acquiesced (Quinones, 2015).

In 1961, member states of the United Nations adopted the *Single Convention on Narcotic Drugs*, declaring that the medical use of narcotic drugs was indispensable for pain relief and recommending that countries ensure adequate provision of narcotic drugs for medical use (Lande, 1962). It would be another 25 years before prescription opioids garnered serious medical attention since throughout the later part of the 20th century most medical professionals in the United States believed that the long-term use of opioids to treat chronic pain was contraindicated by the risk of addiction, increased disability, and diminishing efficacy over time (Rosenblum, Marsch, Joseph, & Portenoy, 2008). Medical practice patterns remained largely aligned with those beliefs until intensive marketing strategies were used to change opinion and practice (Van Zee, 2009).

Two articles published in medical journals in the 1980s were used by industry to reverse medical concerns and to advance safety claims (Van Zee, 2009). The first was a one-paragraph opinion piece on the use of opioids for acute pain;

it was not a formal study (Porter & Jick, 1980). The second concerned opioid use for chronic pain and was based on a small sample of highly controlled subjects in a particular hospital setting (Portenoy & Foley, 1986). Both articles suggested that concerns related to prescription opioid addiction might not be as serious a problem as once thought. At about the same time, the World Health Organization elevated attention to the under-treatment of postoperative pain and cancer pain in 1986 with the publication of a Cancer Pain Monograph that focused on a small number of inexpensive drugs, including morphine, for cancer pain (World Health Organization, 1986).

Although both of the 1980s articles were later cited by industry representatives to justify greater use of opioid medications and to downplay addiction concerns, there was nothing inherently "wrong" with these early publications; they did not portend to be more than they were. Even though the addictive properties of opioids were well known by physicians, pharmacists, and pharmaceutical companies world wide, including companies like Merck and Bayer, by the start of the 1990s, there were no population-level studies that established a safety risk between chronic use of pharmaceutical opioids and addiction. The two articles were offered less as evidence of safety to prescribers than a veil of legitimacy, given that a critical reading of either article would reveal that their findings were not scientifically rigorous. As such, in the absence of a randomized controlled trial that demonstrated risk, it was the use of these articles that helped to confer presumed safety on pharmaceutical opioids.

By the mid-1990s, the campaign to eradicate pain had gained momentum. In 1995, the American Pain Society launched an influential "pain as the fifth vital sign" campaign to add evaluation and treatment of pain symptoms to the four vital signs of: body temperature, blood pressure, pulse (heart rate), and breathing rate (respiratory rate) (Campbell, 1996). The Veterans Health Administration (VHA) followed and adopted pain as the fifth vital sign in 1999 (Kerns, Wasse, Ryan, Drake, & Bross, 2000). The Joint Commission (JC) followed shortly by publishing standards for pain management in 2000, emphasizing the need for medical organizations to conduct quantitative assessments of pain as part of accreditation requirements (Phillips, 2000). Even as various policy manifestations of the "War on Drugs" raged through the Nixon, Reagan, Bush (HW), Clinton, and Bush (W), administrations, "illegal" drugs, and not the pharmaceutical industries profiting from addiction, remained the enemy (Whitford & Yates, 2009).

No robust literature on the effectiveness of opioid medications for controlling non-cancer chronic pain emerged during the 1990s that might explain the willingness of governmental and accrediting bodies to endorse greater use of prescription opioids in light of impending addiction and overdose risks. As marketing efforts grew, some researchers suggested that the risk of addiction was slim and that high-risk patients could be identified and managed so that the overall benefits likely mitigated concerns (Aronoff, 2000; Fishman et al., 2000). This framing, combined with a dearth of robust clinical trials proving addictive properties associated with pharmaceutical-grade opioid medications, allowed government and industry to frame the risk of addiction along moral, race, and class lines (Whitford & Yates, 2009).

By 1997, studies began to emerge about the effectiveness of prescription opioids to manage chronic pain, but it would be a few years before a review concluded that opioids may be efficacious for short-term pain relief, but efficacy after 16 weeks was unclear (Martell et al., 2007). In the meantime, industry carefully crafted the marketing of its new opioid medications to target specific demographics far away from the "street" opioids that Nixon had linked to urban Black and Brown people two decades earlier (Van Zee, 2009). By the late 1990s, prescribing analgesics for non-cancer pain had become common practice (Ashburn & Staats, 1999), and pharmaceutical companies were at the center of prescription opioid promotion.

For example, the Sackler family's Purdue Pharma introduced MS Contin, a morphine sulfate drug for pain in 1987 (U.S. Food and Drug Administration, 2020), just after the WHO's Pain Monograph was published. By 1990, MS Contin's potential for abuse and serious risks of addiction had been established (Crews & Denson, 1990). Nevertheless, Purdue Pharma introduced and aggressively marketed a new opioid, OxyContin (oxycodone hydrochloride) in 1996, even as Purdue's own 1995 testing demonstrated that 68% of the oxycodone could be extracted from an OxyContin tablet when crushed. That disclosure was submitted to the FDA in 1995 before OxyContin was approved and released to the public (Purdue Pharma, 1995). Despite this knowledge of its susceptibility to tampering and potential abuse, the FDA approved and Purdue promoted OxyContin. From 1997 to 2002, OxyContin prescriptions increased from 670,000 to 6.2 million (Jones et al., 2018), and sales grew from $48 million in 1996 to almost $1.1 billion in 2000 (Purdue Pharma, 2002).

Downplaying Risk and Creating Acceptability

Although OxyContin was a new formulation, it did not outperform other pain medications (Hale et al., 1999). Its main advantage appeared to be its extended release formulation (12 hours). To sell the new formulation, Purdue Pharma had to create demand. To create demand, they downplayed risk (Van Zee, 2009). Purdue "aggressively" promoted the use of opioids for non-malignant pain (Purdue Pharma, 2002). Strategies included:

- From 1996 to 2001, Purdue Pharma trained more than 5,000 physicians, pharmacists, and nurses at all-expenses-paid symposia for its national speakers' bureau. Although medical providers sometimes dismiss the role that such incentives have on their prescribing behaviors, research suggests that paying and rewarding physicians actually positively influences their prescribing behaviors (Orlowski & Wateska, 1992).
- The company created a prescriber database that targeted the highest prescribers across the country.
- It developed a lucrative bonus system for sales representatives. In 2001, Purdue paid $40 million in incentive bonuses to its sales representatives (U.S. General Accounting Office, 2003).
- From 1996 to 2001, Purdue Pharma more than doubled its sales force from 318 sales representatives to 671.
- The company started a new initiator coupon program for a free, limited-time prescription for a 7- to 30-day supply. Approximately 34,000 coupons were redeemed nationally.
- The company gave away lots of free promotional materials (swag)—including fishing hats and stuffed animals (U.S. General Accounting Office, 2003).

By 2003, nearly half of all physicians prescribing OxyContin worked in primary care (U.S. General Accounting Office, 2003). Perdue representatives told prescribers that the risk for developing dependence was less than 1% for those who initiated opioids (Meier, 2003), even though by 1997, the scientific literature offered percentages that ranged from 1% to 27% among those who had an opioid exposure (Højsted & Sjøgren, 2007).

In contrast to Nixon's framing, the marketing and targeting of OxyContin was heavily rural and largely White. From 1998 through 2000, in states like Maine, West Virginia, eastern Kentucky, southwestern Virginia, and Alabama, hydrocodone and oxycodone were prescribed 2.5 to 5.0 times more than the national average (Drug Enforcement Administration, 2002). As prescription rates in these states went up, so did the cases of hepatitis C and the demand for opioid treatment (Van Zee, 2009). In eastern Kentucky, for example, over a 6-year period (from 1995 to 2001), there was a 500% increase in the number of patients entering methadone maintenance treatment programs, approximately 75% of whom were OxyContin dependent (Van Zee, 2009).

The campaign to make opioid prescriptions for non-cancer pain acceptable had worked. By 2004, OxyContin had become the most prevalent prescription opioid abused in the United States (Cicero, Inciardi, & Muñoz, 2005). More broadly, the campaign to make prescription opioids acceptable among the rural poor had taken hold across the country and was reflected in higher national opioid prescription rates among Medicaid beneficiaries from at least 2006–2015 (Guy, 2017). For example, Washington State analyzed overdose deaths involving prescription opioids during 2004–2007. Researchers found that 1,668 persons died from prescription opioid-related overdoses during the period (6.4 deaths per 100,000 per year); 45.4% of deaths were among persons enrolled in Medicaid (CDC, 2009).

As an indication of the disproportionate mortality among poor people, one might note that the age-adjusted rate of opioid overdose death was 30.8 per 100,000 in the Medicaid-enrolled population, compared with 4.0 per 100,000 in the non-Medicaid population. This suggests that Medicaid-eligible patients had an age-adjusted relative risk of 5.7, meaning that Medicaid patients had odds of dying from an overdose nearly 6 times greater than those with private insurance (CDC, 2009). Medicaid is a public program for eligible poor people funded by a combination of Federal and State tax dollars.

Some have suggested that the targeting of prescription opioids to rural, largely White communities has been protective for communities of color (Frakt & Monkovic, 2019). Given the opioid use disorder and mortality data from the 1970s, and decades-long drug enforcement practices that have targeted poor communities and communities of color going at least as far back as the Nixon administration, to suggest that reduced access to pain medication was somehow "protective" would seem unwarranted. Rather, one might consider how the "War on Drugs" impacted communities of color, how Big Pharma's focus on rural communities impacted poor White communities, and whether the intentional marketing to rural Whites was created, at least in part, as a racial foil to Nixon's linking of narcotics and "street crime" to create cognitive separation between "street" opioids (narcotics) and pharmaceutical grade opioids. Recent legal disclosures that the pharmaceutical industry and personal profits drove the marketing decisions to focus on rural communities and not a desire to protect a particular racial/ethnic or economic population suggest that protecting any community was an unlikely motivator (Hoffman, 2019). Indeed, institutionalized racial policies are rarely protective (Krieger, 2012).

Turning

In what would signal a turning point for the opioid industry, on May 10, 2007, Purdue Frederick Company Inc., and three company executives pled guilty to criminal charges of misbranding OxyContin by claiming that it was less addictive and less subject to abuse and diversion than other opioids (Meier, 2007). Additional lawsuits followed.

Purdue Pharma shares a large portion of responsibility for the prescription opioid epidemic. However, (1) the addictive properties of opioids have been known for centuries; (2) having had years of chemistry and biology courses, physicians and pharmacists are highly trained; (3) the FDA holds official regulatory oversight over medications; (4) the DEA can legally curtail the supply of controlled pharmaceutical substances; and (5) the leading pharmaceutical companies hire the best talent available. There is plenty of responsibility to be shared.

Following the 2007 court decision, an abuse-deterrent formulation of OxyContin was introduced in 2010 that was more difficult to solubilize or crush. The formulation was marketed to discourage abuse through injection and inhalation (Cicero, Ellis, & Surratt, 2012). The new formulation was effective at reducing abuse of OxyContin, but it was also associated with a host of negative consequences. From 2008–2012, for example, the original OxyContin had been a primary drug of abuse before the release of the 2010 formulation among 36% of respondents of 2,500 surveyed individuals who entered substance abuse treatment for whom a prescription opioid was the primary drug of abuse. The number dropped to 13% 21 months later, while the use of other opioids, including fentanyl, increased from 20% to 32%. Of all opioids used to "get high in the past 30 days at least once," OxyContin fell from 47% of respondents to 30% while heroin use nearly doubled (Cicero et al., 2012).

> "It is important to note that there was no evidence that OxyContin abusers ceased their drug abuse as a result of the abuse-deterrent formulation. Rather, it appears that they simply shifted their drug of choice."
>
> **Cicero, Ellis, & Surratt** (2012)

Although 24% of the surveyed respondents managed to compromise the tamper-resistant properties of the abuse-deterrent OxyContin formulation, a far greater number—66%—switched to another opioid, with "heroin" as the most common response. One of the respondents stated: "Most people that I know don't use OxyContin to get high anymore. They have moved on to heroin [because] it is easier to use, much cheaper, and easily available." The respondent, like the authors of the study, observed that those who have opioid dependence will likely switch to an alternative form that is cheaper and readily available (Cicero et al., 2012).

As described earlier in this chapter, the presence of fentanyl in many heroin and other drug (e.g. cocaine) products creates greater risk for opioid-related overdose and death. Given the extent of OxyContin use before the formulation changed, it is possible that the switch in the OxyContin formulation contributed to an increase in heroin/fentanyl deaths as those who had become dependent on the previous formulation sought out heroin. Changes in supply and formulation of prescription opioid medications can have widespread health consequences, as do industry marketing strategies and governmental policies (Posner, 2020).

White Race and Prescriptions

As described above, analgesics were heavily marketed in rural, largely White areas. Dramatic increases in opioid overdose deaths in those areas quickly followed, such that by 2010 White prescription opioid overdose deaths were twice that of Blacks. The mortality rates were so extensive that the CDC suggested that overdoses were at the center of reduced life expectancy in the population (Redfield, 2018), although others have argued that pointing to a single factor among one portion of the population is an oversimplification of longer trends (Muennig, Reynolds, Fink, Zafari, & Geronimus, 2018).

We know that African Americans received fewer prescriptions, but the prescription differential was not just about where pharmaceutical companies chose to market products (Swift et al., 2019). African Americans received fewer opioid prescriptions, some researchers think, because many medical providers restricted access because they wrongly believed that Black and Brown patients were:

1. More likely to become addicted to the drugs
2. More likely to sell the drugs
3. Had a higher pain threshold than White people
4. Less deserving of pain relief (Frakt & Monkovic, 2019).

Since African Americans received fewer prescriptions, fewer died of a related overdose (Alexander et al., 2018). However, many Black and Brown patients likely endured debilitating pain from cancer and other conditions in the absence of indicated pain medication.

As the country started to take notice of escalating opioid-related mortality among Whites, medicine, public health, criminal justice, the media and other interests created important narratives framing opioid use disorders as a biological disease while expanding treatment resources—an approach that was far removed from the criminalizing narratives that have historically described narcotic use by people of color (Netherland & Hansen, 2017). The emerging treatment-centric, public health focused approach to opioid use disorders is a long overdue change to public policy. However, it is hard to overstate the negative economic, educational, and public health impact that the "War on Drugs" has had on poor people, and disproportionately on communities of color (Iguchi, Bell, Ramchand, & Fain, 2005; Moore & Elkavich, 2008; Weidner & Schultz, 2019). See **Figure 2-3**.

State and Federal governments' focus of late has been to reduce pharmaceutical opioid supplies by reigning in opioid prescriptions and to increase harm reduction intervention (naloxone) and treatment strategies (Christie et al., 2017). Even as policies bend toward a "gentler," more public health prevention and treatment approach, nearly 300,000 people are held in state and federal prisons in the United States for drug-law violations, up from less than 25,000 in 1980 (Gelb et al., 2018). As of January of 2021, 46.3% of inmates in federal prisons were there on drug-related crimes (Federal Bureau of Prisons, 2021).

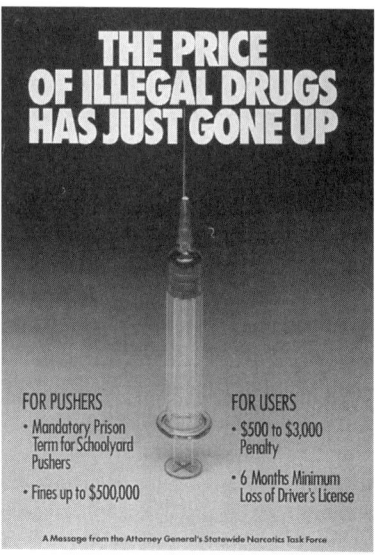

Figure 2-3 The Price of Illegal Drugs Has Just Gone Up.

National Library of Medicine. Retrieved from https://collections.nlm.nih.gov/catalog/nlm:nlmuid-101437971-img

Beyond Black and White

The sale and use of opioids in the United States has long been racialized. However, there is danger of viewing the most recent opioid epidemic through a lens that reflects only a Black/White dichotomy. Although the subsequent text begins to offer a glimpse of the impact of opioids on other communities, there is a tendency, especially with large data sets, to group race and ethnicity by macro-categories. This aggregation obscures important differences by region and country of origin, immigration status, and other important considerations (González Burchard et al., 2005; Wu et al., 2013).

For the following, imperfect for the reasons just identified, Hispanic or Latinx refers to a person of Cuban, Mexican, Puerto Rican, South or Central American, or other Spanish culture or origin regardless of race (Ennis, Rios-Vargas, & Albert, 2011). Although rates of substance use disorders for "illicit" drugs and need for substance use disorder treatment are comparable to other racial/ethnic groups, having experienced discrimination and acculturation have been associated with greater odds of opioid use disorders among Hispanics and Latinx (Blanco et al., 2013; Verissimo, Grella, Amaro, & Gee, 2014). Historically, many poor Hispanic and Latinx peoples have not had access to medical care services given that health insurance is expensive and not readily available through many sectors that have historically employed larger numbers of Hispanic and Latinx peoples (e.g. farming, construction, domestic labor). In addition, among the high numbers of community members who have been employed in production and construction sectors with higher risk of labor-based injuries (U.S. Bureau of Labor Statistics, 2019), identification of pain symptoms and perception of need by the medical community have not always aligned (Hollingshead, Ashburn-Nardo, Stewart, & Hirsh, 2016; Nguyen, Ugarte, Fuller, Haas, & Portenoy, 2005). Hispanic/Latinx clients have initiated treatment more often for heroin use and are referred to treatment more often by the criminal justice system than Whites (Reif, Horgan, & Ritter, 2008). However, like African Americans, Hispanic/Latinx peoples have significantly lower rates of completing specialty care substance disorder treatment (Guerrero et al., 2013), and less access to buprenorphine through physicians' outpatient office-based substance use disorder treatment services than Whites (Lagisetty, Ross, Bohnert, Clay, & Maust, 2019).

The National Survey of Drug Use and Health suggests that American-Indian/Alaskan Natives (AI/AN) may have slightly higher substance use rates than other groups. However, from 2015–2018, across all AI/AN age groups, there were no significant changes in prescription opioid misuse, initiation of misuse, or opioid use disorders. Similarly, there were no significant changes in heroin use initiation, use, or use disorders (Substance Abuse and Mental Health Services Administration [SAMHSA], 2019).

Like non-Hispanic Whites, the opioid overdose mortality rate among AI/AN has risen over the last two decades. In 1999, the age-adjusted annual opioid mortality rate among AI/AN was 2.9 deaths per 100,000; by 2016, that rate had risen to 13.9 per 100,000. Data aggregation can mask wide variation within a state (and by tribe). For example, the Minnesota AI/AN mortality rate was 47.6 per 100,000, while the non-Hispanic White rate was 7.3 per 100,000 in 2016, while states like Arizona and New Mexico reported AI rates under 6 per 100,000 (Tipps, Buzzard, & McDougall, 2018).

The funding and delivery of health care for AI/AN communities constitutes a complicated matrix of Indian Health Service (IHS) and self-determination contracts operating independent tribal health services. In 2019, the IHS reported serving 2.56 million AI/NA across 573 federally recognized Tribes in 37 states (IHS, 2020). In 2019, IHS operated 24 hospitals and 50 health centers while tribes managed 22 hospitals and 285 health centers (IHS, 2020). Both IHS and tribal health centers can offer MOUD. Like states, Tribes, as sovereign nations, can use their criminal and civil jurisdiction to craft specific policy responses including wellness courts and lawsuits against opioid manufacturers.

Starting in 2015, the IHS initiated several measures to reduce overdose deaths, including the promotion and distribution of naloxone, required opioid training for all prescribers, and in 2016, mandated that providers check states' Prescription Drug Monitoring Program databases prior to prescribing and dispensing opioids longer than seven days (Katzman et al., 2016; Tipps et al., 2018). The total number of individuals receiving pharmacotherapy (buprenorphine or methadone) for an opioid use disorder has grown steadily from 2016 among AI/NA patients with an opioid use disorder, suggesting that access to medication has increased (SAMHSA, 2019). Although access is improving, there can be challenges melding traditional healing practices with "evidence-based" substance use disorder treatment, especially when such programs have not been developed within AI/NA communities. Often, "evidence-based" treatment modalities are rooted in paradigms that are inconsistent with traditional cultures, but U.S. federal policies may preclude cost reimbursement for traditional methodologies (Novins et al., 2011; Venner et al., 2018).

The National Survey of Drug Use and Health suggests that Asian/Pacific Islanders have tended to have some of the lowest opioid use rates, (although there appears to be some variation between Asian/Pacific Islanders groups) (Wu et al., 2013). Although treatment admission rates have been increasing (Sahker, Yeung, Garrison, Park, & Arndt, 2017), Asian Americans/Pacific Islanders have the lowest rates of treatment initiation among those with an opioid use disorder compared with Whites (Wu, Zhu, & Swartz, 2016). Cultural barriers related to shame, racial discrimination, and access to affordable health insurance have been suggested as reasons for low treatment entry (Fong & Tsuang, 2007; Masson et al., 2013).

The United States invaded Afghanistan in 2001 and Iraq in 2003. Compared with previous wars, both conflicts saw a significant increase in injuries to the head and neck (Hoencamp et al., 2014). While there were relatively fewer deaths compared with previous wars, serious injuries increased along with the need to manage pain after combat trauma, during acute medical treatment, and throughout rehabilitation (Clark, Bair, Buckenmaier, Gironda, & Walker, 2007). Military physicians wrote nearly 3.8 million prescriptions for pain medication in 2009, more than four times the number of prescriptions written in 2001 (Morden, Oster, & O'Brien, 2013).

Following guidance from the Veterans Health Administration (Lin et al., 2017; Management of Opioid Therapy for Chronic Pain Working Group, 2010), the number of Veterans Health Administration patients who received a prescription opioid within 3 months before death declined from 54% in 2010 to 26% in 2016 (Lin et al., 2019). During the same period, the rate of opioid overdose among veterans increased from 14.5 (per 100,000 person-years) in 2010 to 21.1 (per 100,000 person-years) in 2016. Although there was a decline in methadone overdose and no change in natural/semisynthetic opioid overdose rate, the synthetic opioid overdose rate and heroin overdose rate increased substantially (Lin et al., 2019).

State Interventions

Prescription drug monitoring programs (PDMP) use an electronic database to track controlled substance prescriptions in a state. These secure data systems allow both those who write and those who fill the prescription to check a patient's history to see if there are multiple opioid prescriptions or other indications of irregularities. The first PDMP program began in New York State in 1918 to monitor prescriptions for cocaine, codeine, heroin, morphine, and opium (Bulloch, 2018). Although PDMPs have existed for years to monitor diversion and misuse, prescriber participation in most PDMP programs was often voluntary.

Forty-nine of the 50 states (Missouri is the exception) have a PDMP. The requirements for PDMPs vary. Some are completely voluntary (n = 7), others require just the prescriber to consult the database before issuing a prescription for a controlled substance (n = 27), while the remaining (n = 19) require that both prescribers and dispensers check the data bases (Prescription Drug Monitoring Program Technical Assistance and Training Program, 2019). Mandates can often take one of two forms: "registration mandates" require prescribers to register and to query a database prior to prescribing opioids; "use mandates" allow prescribers' delegates (e.g., nurses) to check the PDMP database (Haffajee, Jena, & Weiner, 2015).

The public health impact of PDMP mandates appears mixed. Some PDMP mandates are associated with reductions in the total opioid dosage prescribed and number of opioid prescriptions filled but are less consistently associated with reductions in the number of patients prescribed opioids (Haffajee et al., 2018). In New York State, a study examining the adoption of a PDMP mandate in 2013 found that although the number of prescriptions appeared to have declined, MMEs appear to have increased after adoption of the mandate. The study found that the prescription opioid overdose rate in New York did not increase significantly after the mandate (note: it also did not decrease), but the rate of heroin overdoses sharply increased. The study's authors suggest that the increase could be attributable either to people turning to heroin when the prescription opioid supply constricted or to increased fentanyl within the heroin supply (Brown et al., 2017).

PDMPs are not the only state-level intervention. Several states that experienced rapid increases in inappropriate opioid prescribing from doctors, clinics, or pharmacies (colloquially known as "pill mills") saw reductions in opioid prescriptions and diversions as state legislatures tightened regulations on "pill mills." "Pill mills" are quick-stop opioid prescribing shops that proliferated across the country, but disproportionately in the South (Lyapustina et al., 2016; Surratt et al., 2014).

Healthcare Implications

Access to substance use disorder treatment is often associated with possessing health insurance and health insurance in the United States is still (with some exceptions like federally supported Medicare for elders or Medicaid for the poor) often a benefit extended through employment (Becker et al., 2008; Maclean & Saloner, 2019). The Affordable Care Act (ACA) broadened access to health insurance and created significant reductions in the number of people without insurance across all major racial groups. In addition, the insurance coverage gaps between Whites and non-Whites (before the ACA, Whites had higher rates of health insurance-often related to higher employment rates and job sector affiliations) shrank for all major groups. Asian Americans, Native Hawaiians, and Pacific Islanders saw the insurance coverage disparity with Whites disappear entirely under the ACA (Park et al., 2018).

A large study of integrated care (combining primary medical and mental health care) within the Kaiser Permanente health system found that patients with substance use disorders, particularly those with opioid use disorders, had significantly greater odds of having comorbid health conditions (asthma, diabetes, etc.) than patients without substance use disorders. The significantly higher rate of comorbid conditions suggests an opportunity for providers to use an integrated care model to treat and manage multiple conditions, including substance use disorders, among their patient populations (Bahorik, Satre, Kline-Simon, Weisner, & Campbell, 2017).

Integrated care uses a team of medical and mental health professionals to address both medical and mental health/substance use disorders in primary care (Burnam & Watkins, 2006). While there are different strategies (Korthuis et al., 2017), a coordinated, integrated, patient-centered approach is at the center of most models (Kringos, Boerma, Hutchinson, van der Zee, & Groenewegen, 2010). Variations in models and measures can present challenges to assessing the effectiveness of integrated care, which can also be known as collaborative care, but it is widely praised and adopted (Crowley & Kirschner, 2015; Lagisetty et al., 2017). SAMHSA and the Health Services and Research Administration have partnered to offer resources, including training and technical assistance to support integrated care (SAMHSA, 2017).

For the first time, on June 9, 2020, the United States Preventive Services Task Force (USPSTF) published a final recommendation statement on the effectiveness of screening for unhealthy drug use in primary care. The Task Force recommended that primary care clinicians ask adults about their drug use and connect people who have a problem with substance use disorder treatment (Krist et al., 2020). The recommendation could increase early opioid use detection and treatment access. Although relatively few people find their way to a specialty care mental health provider, most people see a physician on a regular basis (CDC, 2017).

The USPSTF recommendation increases the chances that a disorder may be detected before other problems (e.g., HCV or HIV infection) manifest. In addition, because it is a level "B" recommendation, the patient cannot be charged a co-payment for the screening under current Affordable Care Act provisions (Kaiser Family Foundation, 2015). Although the new USPSTF recommendation offers promise for earlier detection and greater treatment access, there are also challenges. Stigma has long been associated with opioid use disorders (Acker, 1993). Movement away from a criminal justice approach to substance use disorders toward a disease model (McLellan, Lewis, O'Brien, & Kleber, 2000), including a focus on the neurological underpinnings of substance use disorders, has helped to counter the morality narrative (Volkow, Koob, & McLellan, 2016), but others have been critical of framing substance use disorders as a brain disease to reduce stigma, in part because disease itself is stigmatized (Hammer et al., 2013). There are also pragmatic limitations. It is worth noting that if primary care physicians were to conduct all recommended patient screenings, it would add more than seven hours a day to their workday (Yarnall, Pollak, Østbye, Krause, & Michener, 2003).

In addition, medicine can be slow to change old practice patterns to adopt evidence-based practices—sometimes up to 17 years (Morris, Wooding, & Grant, 2011). In the case of substance use disorders, for example, screening for harmful alcohol use has been recommended by the USPSTF since 2004 (USPSTF, 2004). However, wide spread screening has generally not been fully adopted in primary care (Haley, Moscou, Murray, Rieckmann, & Wells, 2019). Although alcohol abuse is far more common than opioid use and upward of 38 million people drink to excess, fewer than 20% of patients speak with their doctor, nurse, or other health professional about their drinking (CDC, 2014).

Structural issues, such as a lack of institutional and mental health support have been identified as barriers to buprenorphine treatment in primary care (Hutchinson, Catlin, Andrilla, Baldwin, & Rosenblatt, 2014), while expansions to nursing responsibilities and support has increased patient uptake (LaBelle, Han, Bergeron, & Samet, 2016). In addition, a systematic review suggests that some health professionals may hold negative attitudes about patients with substance use disorders, although those with more professional experience with substance use disorders reported more positive attitudes (van Boekel et al., 2013). Stated reasons for negative attitudes include safety concerns, perceived manipulation, aggression, rudeness, and patients' lack of motivation. In addition, causal attribution, when providers believe patients should have greater control over their disease, has been associated with greater intolerance of patients with substance use disorders (Livingston, Milne, Fang, & Amari, 2012). And while training can improve provider engagement (Hammer et al., 2013), organizational capacity, including appropriate support systems, staffing, and funding are associated with effective treatment within integrated care (Kaplan et al., 2010; Knudsen, Abraham, & Oser, 2011).

Discussion Questions

1. Does the CDC miss any trends in its assertion that the current opioid epidemic can be described in three waves? If yes, please describe.
2. Why might someone who has grown dependent on opioids switch from their preferred opioid compound to a different opioid? What are the potential health implications of such a substitution?
3. Identify the historical and current contributing factors that would allow the current opioid epidemic to be considered iatrogenic? What factors argue against such a characterization?
4. How does race factor into how prescription opioids were marketed?
5. How has race or class influenced how the opioid epidemic has been depicted in the media and the focus of interventions in this most recent iteration? What are the differences between now and the late 1960s/ early 1970s?
6. Why were most PDMPs not associated with reductions in opioid mortality?
7. Explain why opioid overdoses are often treated as acute events when patients are brought to hospitals and not as a symptom of a chronic condition?

References

Acker, C. J. (1993). Stigma or legitimation? A historical examination of the social potentials of addiction disease models. *Journal of Psychoactive Drugs, 25*(3), 193–205. doi:10.1080/027910 72.1993.10472271

Alexander, M. J., Kiang, M. V., & Barbieri, M. (2018). Trends in black and white opioid mortality in the United States, 1979–2015. *Epidemiology (Cambridge, Mass.), 29*(5), 707–715. doi:10.1097 /EDE.0000000000000858

Allen, B., Nolan, M. L., Kunins, H. V., & Paone, D. (2019). Racial differences in opioid overdose deaths in New York City, 2017. *JAMA Internal Medicine, 179*(4), 576–578. doi:10.1001 /jamainternmed.2018.7700

Aronoff, G. M. (2000). Opioids in chronic pain management:Is there a significant risk of addiction? *Current Review of Pain, 4*(2), 112–121. doi:10.1007/s11916-000-0044-0

Ashburn, M. A., & Staats, P. S. (1999). Management of chronic pain. *The Lancet, 353*(9167), 1865–1869. doi:10.1016/S0140-6736(99)04088-X

Bahorik, A. L., Satre, D. D., Kline-Simon, A. H., Weisner, C. M., & Campbell, C. I. (2017). Alcohol, cannabis, and opioid use disorders, and disease burden in an integrated healthcare system. *Journal of Addiction Medicine, 11*(1), 39. doi:10.1097/ADM.0000000000000260

Baum, D. (2016, April). Legalize it all. *Harper's Magazine.* Retrieved from https://harpers.org/archive /2016/04/legalize-it-all

Bebinger, M. (2017a). *As the opium trade boomed in the 1800s, Boston doctors raised addiction concerns.* Retrieved from https://www.wbur.org/commonhealth/2017/07/31/opium-boston-history

Bebinger, M. (2017b). *How profits from opium shaped 19th-century Boston.* Retrieved from https:// www.wbur.org/commonhealth/2017/08/01/opium-history-addiction

Becker, W. C., Fiellin, D. A., Merrill, J. O., Schulman, B., Finkelstein, R., Olsen, Y., & Busch, S. H. (2008). Opioid use disorder in the United States: Insurance status and treatment access. *Drug and Alcohol Dependence, 94*(1), 207–213. doi:10.1016/j.drugalcdep.2007.11.018

Blanco, C., Morcillo, C., Alegría, M., Dedios, M. C., Fernández-Navarro, P., Regincos, R., & Wang, S. (2013). Acculturation and drug use disorders among Hispanics in the U.S. *Journal of Psychiatric Research, 47*(2), 226–232. doi:10.1016/j.jpsychires.2012.09.019

Brown, R., Riley, M. R., Ulrich, L., Kraly, E. P., Jenkins, P., Krupa, N. L., & Gadomski, A. (2017). Impact of New York prescription drug monitoring program, I-STOP, on statewide overdose morbidity. *Drug and Alcohol Dependence, 178*, 348–354. doi:10.1016/j.drugalcdep.2017.05.023

Bulloch, M. (2018). The evolution of the PDMP. Retrieved from https://www.pharmacytimes.com /contributor/marilyn-bulloch-pharmd-bcps/2018/07/the-evolution-of-the-pdmp

Burnam, M. A., & Watkins, K. E. (2006). Substance abuse with mental disorders: specialized public systems and integrated care. *Health Affairs, 25*(3), 648–658. doi:10.1377/hlthaff.25.3.648

Campbell, J. N. (1996). *APS 1995 presidential address.* Pain Forum. 5:85–88.

Centers for Disease Control and Prevention. (2017). *Ambulatory care use and physician office visits.* Retrieved from https://www.cdc.gov/nchs/fastats/physician-visits.htm

Centers for Disease Control and Prevention. (2020). Understanding the epidemic. Retrieved from https://www.cdc.gov/drugoverdose/epidemic

Centers for Disease Control and Prevention. (2009). Overdose deaths involving prescription opioids among Medicaid enrollees—Washington, 2004–2007. *Morbidity and Mortality Weekly Report, 58*(42), 1171–1175. Retrieved from https://www.cdc.gov/mmwr/preview/mmwrhtml /mm5842a1.htm

Centers for Disease Control Prevention. (2014). Alcohol screening and counseling: An effective but underused health service. Retrieved from https://www.cdc.gov/vitalsigns/alcohol-screening -counseling/index.html

Christie, C., Baker, C., Cooper, R., Kennedy, P. J., Madras, B., & Bondi, P. (2017). *The president's commission on combating drug addiction and the opioid crisis.* Washington, DC: U.S. Government Printing Office. Retrieved from https://www.whitehouse.gov/sites/whitehouse.gov/files/images /Final_Report_Draft_11-15-2017.pdf

Cicero, T. J., Ellis, M. S., & Surratt, H. L. (2012). Effect of abuse-deterrent formulation of OxyContin. *The New England Journal of Medicine, 367*(2), 187–189. doi:10.1056/NEJMc1204141

Cicero, T. J., Inciardi, J. A., & Muñoz, A. (2005). Trends in abuse of OxyContin® and other opioid analgesics in the United States: 2002–2004. *The Journal of Pain, 6*(10), 662–672. doi:10.1016/j .jpain.2005.05.004

Clark, M. E., Bair, M. J., Buckenmaier, C. C., III, Gironda, R. J., & Walker, R. L. (2007). Pain and combat injuries in soldiers returning from Operations Enduring Freedom and Iraqi Freedom: Implications for research and practice. *Journal of Rehabilitation Research & Development, 44*(2), 179–194. doi:10.1682/jrrd.2006.05.0057

Council of Economic Advisors. (2017). *The Underestimated Cost of the Opioid Crisis.* Retrieved from https://www.whitehouse.gov/sites/whitehouse.gov/files/images/The%20Underestimated%20 Cost%20of%20the%20Opioid%20Crisis.pdf

Crews, J. C., & Denson, D. D. (1990). Recovery of morphine from a controlled-release preparation: A source of opioid abuse. *Cancer, 66*(12), 2642–2644. doi:10.1002/1097 -0142(19901215)66:12<2642::aid-cncr2820661229>3.0.co;2-b

Crowley, R. A., & Kirschner, N. (2015). The integration of care for mental health, substance abuse, and other behavioral health conditions into primary care: Executive summary of an American College of Physicians position paper. *Annals of Internal Medicine, 163*(4), 298–299. doi:10.7326 /M15-0510

Drug Enforcement Administration. (2002). *States of Alabama, Maine, Kentucky, Virginia, and West Virginia Drug Profile by County—OxyContin, Oxycodone (Excluding OxyContin), and Hydrocodone—2000.* Washington, DC: U.S. Department of Justice.

Drug Enforcement Administration. (2015). *National drug threat assessment summary 2014.* (Pub. no. DEA-DCT-DIR-002–15). Washington, DC: U.S. Department of Justice. Retrieved from https:// www.dea.gov/documents/2014/11/01/2014-national-drug-threat-assessment

Ennis, S., Rios-Vargas, M., & Albert, N. (2011). The Hispanic population: 2010. *2010 Census Briefs.* Retrieved from https://www2.census.gov/library/publications/cen2010/briefs/c2010br -04.pdf

Federal Bureau of Prisons. (2021). Offenses. Retrieved from https://www.bop.gov/about/statistics /statistics_inmate_offenses.jsp

Fishman, S. M., Wilsey, B., Yang, J., Reisfield, G. M., Bandman, T. B., & Borsook, D. (2000). Adherence monitoring and drug surveillance in chronic opioid therapy. *Journal of Pain and Symptom Management, 20*(4), 293–307. doi:10.1016/S0885-3924(00)00195-0

Fong, T. W., & Tsuang, J. (2007). Asian-Americans, addictions, and barriers to treatment. *Psychiatry (Edgmont), 4*(11), 51–59.

Frakt, A., & Monkovic, T. (2019, November 25). A 'rare case where racial biases' protected African-Americans. *New York Times*. Retrieved from https://www.nytimes.com/2019/11/25/upshot/opioid-epidemic-blacks.html

Gelb, A., Stevenson, P., Fifield, A., Fuhrman, M., Bennet, L., Horowitz, J., & Boradus, E. (2018). More imprisonment does not reduce state drug problems. *PEW Issue Brief*. Retrieved from https://www.pewtrusts.org/en/research-and-analysis/issue-briefs/2018/03/more-imprisonment-does-not-reduce-state-drug-problems

González Burchard, E., Borrell, L. N., Choudhry, S., Naqvi, M., Tsai, H.-J., Rodriguez-Santana, J. R., . . . Risch, N. (2005). Latino populations: A unique opportunity for the study of race, genetics, and social environment in epidemiological research. *American Journal of Public Health, 95*(12), 2161–2168. doi:10.2105/AJPH.2005.068668

Guerrero, E. G., Marsh, J. C., Duan, L., Oh, C., Perron, B., & Lee, B. (2013). Disparities in completion of substance abuse treatment between and within racial and ethnic groups. *Health Services Research, 48*(4), 1450–1467. doi:10.1111/1475-6773.12031

Guy, G. P., Jr., Zhang, K., Bohm, M. K., Losby, J., Lewis, B., Young, R., . . . Dowell, D. (2017). Vital signs: changes in opioid prescribing in the United States, 2006–2015. *Morbidity and Mortality Weekly Report, 66*(26), 697–704. Retrieved from https://www.cdc.gov/mmwr/volumes/66/wr/mm6626a4.htm

Haffajee, R. L., Jena, A. B., & Weiner, S. G. (2015). Mandatory use of prescription drug monitoring programs. *JAMA, 313*(9), 891–892. doi:10.1001/jama.2014.18514

Haffajee, R. L., Mello, M. M., Zhang, F., Zaslavsky, A. M., Larochelle, M. R., & Wharam, J. F. (2018). Four states with robust prescription drug monitoring programs reduced opioid dosages. *Health Affairs, 37*(6), 964–974. doi:10.1377/hlthaff.2017.1321

Hale, M. E., Fleischmann, R., Salzman, R., Wild, J., Iwan, T., Swanton, R. E., . . . Lacouture, P. G. (1999). Efficacy and safety of controlled-release versus immediate-release oxycodone: Randomized, double-blind evaluation in patients with chronic back pain. *The Clinical Journal of Pain, 15*(3), 179–183. doi:10.1097/00002508-199909000-00004

Haley, S. J., Moscou, S., Murray, S., Rieckmann, T., & Wells, K. L. (2019). The availability of alcohol, tobacco and other drug services for adults in New York State community health centers. *Journal of Substance Use, 24*(3), 309–316. doi:10.1080/14659891.2018.1562577

Hammer, R., Dingel, M., Ostergren, J., Partridge, B., McCormick, J., & Koenig, B. A. (2013). Addiction: Current criticism of the brain disease paradigm. *AJOB Neuroscience, 4*(3), 27–32. doi:10.1080/21507740.2013.796328

Hoencamp, R., Vermetten, E., Tan, E. C., Putter, H., Leenen, L. P., & Hamming, J. F. (2014). Systematic review of the prevalence and characteristics of battle casualties from NATO coalition forces in Iraq and Afghanistan. *Injury, 45*(7), 1028–1034. doi:10.1016/j.injury.2014.02.012

Hoffman, J. (2019, August 26). Johnson & Johnson ordered to pay $572 million in landmark opioid trial. *New York Times*. Retrieved from https://www.nytimes.com/2019/08/26/health/oklahoma-opioids-johnson-and-johnson.html

Hollingshead, N. A., Ashburn-Nardo, L., Stewart, J. C., & Hirsh, A. T. (2016). The pain experience of Hispanic Americans: A critical literature review and conceptual model. *The Journal of Pain, 17*(5), 513–528. doi:10.1016/j.jpain.2015.10.022

Hughes, P. H., Barker, N. W., Crawford, G. A., & Jaffe, J. H. (1972). The natural history of a heroin epidemic. *American Journal of Public Health, 62*(7), 995–1001. doi:10.2105/ajph.62.7.995

Hutchinson, E., Catlin, M., Andrilla, C. H. A., Baldwin, L.-M., & Rosenblatt, R. A. (2014). Barriers to primary care physicians prescribing buprenorphine. *The Annals of Family Medicine, 12*(2), 128–133. doi:10.1370/afm.1595

Højsted, J., & Sjøgren, P. (2007). Addiction to opioids in chronic pain patients: A literature review. *European Journal of Pain, 11*(5), 490–518. doi:10.1016/j.ejpain.2006.08.004

Iguchi, M. Y., Bell, J., Ramchand, R. N., & Fain, T. (2005). How criminal system racial disparities may translate into health disparities. *Journal of Health Care for the Poor and Underserved, 16*(4), 48–56. doi:10.1353/hpu.2005.0114

Indian Health Service. (2020). *IHS profile*. Retrieved from https://www.ihs.gov/sites/newsroom/themes/responsive2017/display_objects/documents/factsheets/IHSProfile.pdf

Jones, C. M., Logan, J., Gladden, R. M., & Bohm, M. K. (2015). Vital signs: Demographic and substance use trends among heroin users—United States, 2002–2013. *Morbidity and Mortality Weekly Report, 64*(26), 719–725. Retrieved from https://www.cdc.gov/mmwr/preview/mmwr html/mm6426a3.htm

Jones, M. R., Viswanath, O., Peck, J., Kaye, A. D., Gill, J. S., & Simopoulos, T. T. (2018). A brief history of the opioid epidemic and strategies for pain medicine. *Pain and Therapy, 7*(1), 13–21. doi:10 .1007/s40122-018-0097-6

Kaiser Family Foundation. (2015). Preventive services covered by private health plans under the Affordable Care Act. Retrieved from https://www.kff.org/health-reform/fact-sheet/preventive -services-covered-by-private-health-plans

Kaplan, H. C., Brady, P. W., Dritz, M. C., Hooper, D. K., Linam, W. M., Froehle, C. M., & Margolis, P. (2010). The influence of context on quality improvement success in health care: a systematic review of the literature. *The Milbank Quarterly, 88*(4), 500–559. doi:10.1111/j.1468-0009 .2010.00611.x

Katzman, J. G., Fore, C., Bhatt, S., Greenberg, N., Griffin Salvador, J., Comerci, G. C., . . . Karol, S. (2016). Evaluation of American Indian Health Service training in pain management and opioid substance use disorder. *American Journal of Public Health, 106*(8), 1427–1429. doi:10.2105 /AJPH.2016.303193

Kerns, R., Wasse, L., Ryan, B., Drake, A., & Bross, J. (2000). *Pain as the 5th vital sign toolkit.* (revised ed.). Washington, DC: Veterans Health Administration. Retrieved from https://www.va.gov /painmanagement/docs/pain_as_the_5th_vital_sign_toolkit.pdf

Kerr, P. (1986, September 13). Growth in heroin use ending as city users turn to crack. *New York Times.* Retrieved from https://www.nytimes.com/1986/09/13/nyregion/growth-in-heroin-use-ending-as -city-users-turn-to-crack.html

Knudsen, H. K., Abraham, A. J., & Oser, C. B. (2011). Barriers to the implementation of medication-assisted treatment for substance use disorders: The importance of funding policies and medical infrastructure. *Evaluation and Program Planning, 34*(4), 375–381. doi:10.1016/j .evalprogplan.2011.02.004

Korthuis, P. T., McCarty, D., Weimer, M., Bougatsos, C., Blazina, I., Zakher, B., ... & Chou, R. (2017). Primary care–based models for the treatment of opioid use disorder: A scoping review. *Annals of Internal Medicine, 166*(4), 268–278. doi:10.7326/M16-2149

Krieger, N. (2012). Methods for the scientific study of discrimination and health: An ecosocial approach. *American Journal of Public Health, 102*(5), 936–944. doi:10.2105/AJPH.2011.300544

Kringos, D. S., Boerma, W. G. W., Hutchinson, A., van der Zee, J., & Groenewegen, P. P. (2010). The breadth of primary care: A systematic literature review of its core dimensions. *BMC Health Services Research, 10*(1), 65. doi:10.1186/1472-6963-10-65

Krist, A. H., Davidson, K. W., Mangione, C. M., Barry, M. J., Cabana, M., Caughey, A. B., . . . Epling, J. W. (2020). Screening for unhealthy drug use: US Preventive Services Task Force recommendation statement. *JAMA, 323*(22), 2301–2309. doi:10.1001/jama.2020.8020

LaBelle, C. T., Han, S. C., Bergeron, A., & Samet, J. H. (2016). Office-based opioid treatment with buprenorphine (OBOT-B): Statewide implementation of the Massachusetts Collaborative Care Model in community health centers. *Journal of Substance Abuse Treatment, 60*, 6–13.

Lagisetty, P., Klasa, K., Bush, C., Heisler, M., Chopra, V., & Bohnert, A. (2017). Primary care models for treating opioid use disorders: what actually works? A systematic review. *PloS One, 12*(10), e0186315. doi:10.1371/journal.pone.0186315

Lagisetty, P. A., Ross, R., Bohnert, A., Clay, M., & Maust, D. T. (2019). Buprenorphine treatment divide by race/ethnicity and payment. *JAMA Psychiatry, 76*(9), 979–981. doi:10.1001 /jamapsychiatry.2019.0876

Lande, A. (1962). The single convention on narcotic drugs, 1961. *International Organization, 16*(4), 776–797. doi:10.1017/S0020818300011620

Lin, L. A., Bohnert, A. S. B., Kerns, R. D., Clay, M. A., Ganoczy, D., & Ilgen, M. A. (2017). Impact of the opioid safety initiative on opioid-related prescribing in veterans. *PAIN, 158*(5), 833–839. doi:10.1097/j.pain .0000000000000837. Retrieved from https://journals.lww.com/pain/Fulltext/2017/05000/Impact _of_the_Opioid_Safety_Initiative_on.10.aspx

Lin, L. A., Peltzman, T., McCarthy, J. F., Oliva, E. M., Trafton, J. A., & Bohnert, A. S. (2019). Changing trends in opioid overdose deaths and prescription opioid receipt among veterans. *American Journal of Preventive Medicine, 57*(1), 106–110. doi:10.1016/j.amepre.2019.01.016

Livingston, J. D., Milne, T., Fang, M. L., & Amari, E. (2012). The effectiveness of interventions for reducing stigma related to substance use disorders: A systematic review. *Addiction, 107*(1) 39–50. doi:10.1111/j.1360-0443.2011.03601.x

Lyapustina, T., Rutkow, L., Chang, H.-Y., Daubresse, M., Ramji, A. F., Faul, M., . . . Alexander, G. C. (2016). Effect of a "pill mill" law on opioid prescribing and utilization: The case of Texas. *Drug and Alcohol Dependence, 159*, 190–197. doi:10.1016/j.drugalcdep.2015.12.025

Maclean, J. C., & Saloner, B. (2019). The effect of public insurance expansions on substance use disorder treatment: Evidence from the Affordable Care Act. *Journal of Policy Analysis and Management, 38*(2), 366–393. doi:10.1002/pam.22112

Management of Opioid Therapy for Chronic Pain Working Group. (2010). *VA/DoD clinical practice guideline: Management of opioid therapy for chronic pain.* Washington, DC: US Department of Veterans Affairs, US Department of Defense. Retrieved from https://www.va.gov/painmanagement /docs/cpg_opioidtherapy_fulltext.pdf

Martell, B. A., O'Connor, P. G., Kerns, R. D., Becker, W. C., Morales, K. H., Kosten, T. R., & Fiellin, D. A. (2007). Systematic review: Opioid treatment for chronic back pain: Prevalence, efficacy, and association with addiction. *Annals of Internal Medicine, 146*(2), 116–127. doi:10.7326/0003-4819-146-2-200701160-00006

Masson, C. L., Shopshire, M. S., Sen, S., Hoffman, K. A., Hengl, N. S., Bartolome, J., . . . Iguchi, M. Y. (2013). Possible barriers to enrollment in substance abuse treatment among a diverse sample of Asian Americans and Pacific Islanders: Opinions of treatment clients. *Journal of Substance Abuse Treatment, 44*(3), 309–315. doi:10.1016/j.jsat.2012.08.005

McLellan, A. T., Lewis, D. C., O'Brien, C. P., & Kleber, H. D. (2000). Drug dependence, a chronic medical illness: Implications for treatment, insurance, and outcomes evaluation. *JAMA, 284*(13), 1689–1695. doi:10.1001/jama.284.13.1689

Meier, B. (2003). *Pain killer: A" wonder" drug's trail of addiction and death.* Emmaus, PA: Rodale.

Meier, B. (2007, May 10). In guilty plea, OxyContin maker to pay $600 million. *New York Times.* Retrieved from https://www.nytimes.com/2007/05/10/business/11drug-web.html

Meldrum, M. L. (2016). The ongoing opioid prescription epidemic: Historical context. *American Journal of Public Health, 106*(8), 1365–1366. doi:10.2105/AJPH.2016.303297

Moore, L. D., & Elkavich, A. (2008). Who's using and who's doing time: Incarceration, the war on drugs, and public health. *American Journal of Public Health, 98*(5), 782–786. doi:10.2105/AJPH .2007.126284

Morden, E., Oster, M., & O'Brien, C. P. (Eds.). (2013). *Substance use disorders in the U.S. Armed Forces.* Washington, DC: National Academies Press.

Morris, Z. S., Wooding, S., & Grant, J. (2011). The answer is 17 years, what is the question: Understanding time lags in translational research. *Journal of the Royal Society of Medicine, 104*(12), 510–520. doi:10.1258/jrsm.2011.110180

Muennig, P. A., Reynolds, M., Fink, D. S., Zafari, Z., & Geronimus, A. T. (2018). America's declining well-being, health, and life expectancy: Not just a White problem. *American Journal of Public Health, 108*(12), 1626–1631. doi:10.2105/AJPH.2018.304585

National Center for Health Statistics. (2020). *Wide-ranging online data for epidemiologic research (WONDER).* Retrieved from: http://wonder.cdc.gov.

Netherland, J., & Hansen, H. B. (2016). The war on drugs that wasn't: Wasted whiteness, "dirty doctors," and race in media coverage of prescription opioid misuse. *Culture, Medicine and Psychiatry, 40*(4), 664–686. doi:10.1007/s11013-016-9496-5

Netherland, J., & Hansen, H. (2017). White opioids: Pharmaceutical race and the war on drugs that wasn't. *BioSocieties, 12*(2), 217–238. doi:10.1057/biosoc.2015.46

Nguyen, M., Ugarte, C., Fuller, I., Haas, G., & Portenoy, R. K. (2005). Access to care for chronic pain: Racial and ethnic differences. *The Journal of Pain, 6*(5), 301–314. doi:10.1016/j.jpain.2004.12.008

Nixon, R. (1969). *Special message to the Congress on control of narcotics and dangerous drugs.* Washington, DC: Office of the President. Retrieved from https://www.presidency.ucsb.edu /documents/special-message-the-congress-control-narcotics-and-dangerous-drugs

Novins, D. K., Aarons, G. A., Conti, S. G., Dahlke, D., Daw, R., Fickenscher, A., . . . Centers for American Indian and Alaska Native Health's Substance Abuse Treatment Advisory Board. (2011). Use of the evidence base in substance abuse treatment programs for American Indians and Alaska natives: Pursuing quality in the crucible of practice and policy. *Implementation Science, 6*(1), 63. doi:10.1186/1748-5908-6-63

Office of National Drug Control Policy. (2015). *National drug threat assessment summary 2014.* Washington, DC: Office of the President of the United States. Retrieved from https://www.dea .gov/documents/2014/11/01/2014-national-drug-threat-assessment

Opium eating. (1833). *The Boston Medical and Surgical Journal, 9*(4), 66.

Orlowski, J. P., & Wateska, L. (1992). The effects of pharmaceutical firm enticements on physician prescribing patterns: There's no such thing as a free lunch. *Chest, 102*(1), 270–273. doi:10.1378/chest.102.1.270

Park, J. J., Humble, S., Sommers, B. D., Colditz, G. A., Epstein, A. M., & Koh, H. K. (2018). Health insurance for Asian Americans, Native Hawaiians, and Pacific Islanders under the Affordable Care Act. *JAMA Internal Medicine, 178*(8), 1128–1129. doi:10.1001 /jamainternmed.2018.1476

Pharma. (1995). *New Drug Application to FDA for OxyContin, Pharmacology Review: 'Abuse Liability of Oxycodone.'* Report. Stamford, CT.

Phillips, D. M. (2000). JCAHO pain management standards are unveiled. *JAMA, 284*(4), 428–429. doi:10.1001/jama.284.4.423b

Portenoy, R. K., & Foley, K. M. (1986). Chronic use of opioid analgesics in non-malignant pain: Report of 38 cases. *Pain, 25*(2), 171–186. doi:10.1016/0304-3959(86)90091-6

Porter, J., & Jick, H. (1980). Addiction rare in patients treated with narcotics. *The New England Journal of Medicine, 302*(2), 123. doi:10.1056/nejm198001103020221

Posner, G. (2020). *Pharma: Greed, lies, and the poisoning of America.* New York, NY: Simon & Schuster.

Prescription Drug Monitoring Program Technical Assistance and Training Program. (2020). PDMP Mandatory Query by Prescribers and Dispensers. Retrieved from https://www.pdmpassist.org /pdf/Mandatory_Query_Conditions.pdf

Purdue Pharma. (2002). *OxyContin marketing plan, 2002.* Stamford, CT.

Quinones, S. (2015). *Dreamland: The true tale of America's opiate epidemic.* New York, NY: Bloomsbury Publishing.

Redfield, R. R. (2018). CDC director's media statement on U.S. life expectancy. Retrieved from https://www.cdc.gov/media/releases/2018/s1129-US-life-expectancy.html

Reif, S., Horgan, C. M., & Ritter, G. A. (2008). Hispanics in specialty treatment for substance use disorders. *Journal of Drug Issues, 38*(1), 311–333. doi:10.1177/002204 260803800113

Robins, L. N. (1974). The Vietnam drug user returns. Final report. Special Action Office Monograph, Series A, Number 2, May 1974. Washington, DC: U.S. Government Printing Office. Retrieved from https://files.eric.ed.gov/fulltext/ED134912.pdf

Rosenblum, A., Marsch, L. A., Joseph, H., & Portenoy, R. K. (2008). Opioids and the treatment of chronic pain: Controversies, current status, and future directions. *Experimental and Clinical Psychopharmacology, 16*(5), 405–416. doi:10.1037/a0013628

Sahker, E., Yeung, C. W., Garrison, Y. L., Park, S., & Arndt, S. (2017). Asian American and Pacific Islander substance use treatment admission trends. *Drug and Alcohol Dependence, 171*, 1–8. doi:10.1016/j.drugalcdep.2016.11.022

Seeger, C. (1833). Opium eating. *The Boston Medical and Surgical Journal, 9*(8), 117.

Substance Abuse and Mental Health Services Administration. (2017). SAMHSA-HRSA Center for Integrated Health Solutions. Retrieved from https://www.samhsa.gov/integrated-health -solutions

Substance Abuse and Mental Health Services Administration. (2019). *Key substance use and mental health indicators in the United States: Results from the 2018 National Survey on Drug Use and Health* (HHS Publication No. PEP19-5068, NSDUH Series H-54). Rockville, MD Author. Retrieved from https://www.samhsa.gov/data/sites/default/files/cbhsq-reports/NSDUHNationalFindings Report2018/NSDUHNationalFindingsReport2018.pdf

Substance Abuse and Mental Health Services Administration. (2020). *2018 National Survey on Drug Use and Health: American Indians and Alaska Natives (AI/ANs). [Annual report].* Retrieved from https://www.samhsa.gov/data/report/2018-nsduh-american-indians-and-alaska-natives

Surratt, H. L., O'Grady, C., Kurtz, S. P., Stivers, Y., Cicero, T. J., Dart, R. C., & Chen, M. (2014). Reductions in prescription opioid diversion following recent legislative interventions in Florida. *Pharmacoepidemiology and Drug Safety, 23*(3), 314–320. doi:10.1002/pds.3553

Swift, S. L., Glymour, M. M., Elfassy, T., Lewis, C., Kiefe, C. I., Sidney, S., . . . Zeki Al Hazzouri, A. (2019). Racial discrimination in medical care settings and opioid pain reliever misuse in a U.S. cohort: 1992 to 2015. *PloS One, 14*(12), e0226490. doi:10.1371/journal.pone.0226490

Tipps, R. T., Buzzard, G. T., & McDougall, J. A. (2018). The opioid epidemic in Indian Country. *The Journal of Law, Medicine & Ethics, 46*(2), 422–436. doi:10.1177/1073110518782950

Tricker, E. (2018). Inside the story of America's 19th-century opiate addiction. *Smithsonian Magazine*. Retrieved from https://www.smithsonianmag.com/history/inside-story-americas-19th-century -opiate-addiction-180967673/

U.S. Bureau of Labor Statistics. (2019). Labor force characteristics by race and ethnicity, 2018. *BLS Reports*. Retrieved from https://www.bls.gov/opub/reports/race-and-ethnicity/2018/home.htm

U.S. Food and Drug Administration. (2020). Timeline of Selected FDA Activities and Significant Events Addressing Opioid Misuse and Abuse. Retrieved from https://www.fda.gov/drugs /information-drug-class/timeline-selected-fda-activities-and-significant-events-addressing -opioid-misuse-and-abuse

U.S. General Accounting Office. (2003). *Prescription drugs: OxyContin abuse and diversion and efforts to address the problem: Report to Congressional requesters*. Darby, PA: Diane Publishing.

U.S. Preventive Services Task Force. (2004). Screening and behavioral counseling interventions in primary care to reduce alcohol misuse: Recommendaion statement. *Annals of Internal Medicine, 140*(7), 554–556. doi:10.7326/0003-4819-140-7-200404060-00016

van Boekel, L. C., Brouwers, E. P. M., van Weeghel, J., & Garretsen, H. F. L. (2013). Stigma among health professionals towards patients with substance use disorders and its consequences for healthcare delivery: Systematic review. *Drug and Alcohol Dependence, 131*(1), 23–35. doi:10.1016/j.drugalcdep.2013.02.018

Van Zee, A. (2009). The promotion and marketing of oxycontin: Commercial triumph, public health tragedy. *American Journal of Public Health, 99*(2), 221–227. doi:10.2105/AJPH.2007.131714

Venner, K. L., Donovan, D. M., Campbell, A. N. C., Wendt, D. C., Rieckmann, T., Radin, S. M., . . . Rosa, C. L. (2018). Future directions for medication assisted treatment for opioid use disorder with American Indian/Alaska Natives. *Addictive Behaviors, 86*, 111–117. doi:10.1016/j .addbeh.2018.05.017

Verissimo, A. D. O., Grella, C. E., Amaro, H., & Gee, G. C. (2014). Discrimination and substance use disorders among Latinos: The role of gender, nativity, and ethnicity. *American Journal of Public Health, 104*(8), 1421–1428. doi:10.2105/ajph.2014.302011

Volkow, N. D., Koob, G. F., & McLellan, A. T. (2016). Neurobiologic advances from the brain disease model of addiction. *New England Journal of Medicine, 374*(4), 363–371. doi:10.1056 /NEJMra1511480

Weidner, R. R., & Schultz, J. (2019). Examining the relationship between U.S. incarceration rates and population health at the county level. *SSM-Population Health, 9*. doi:10.1016/j .ssmph.2019.100466

Whitford, A. B., & Yates, J. (2009). *Presidential rhetoric and the public agenda: Constructing the war on drugs*. Baltimore, Maryland: The Johns Hopkins University Press.

World Health Organization. (1986). *Cancer pain relief*. Geneva, Switzerland: Author. Retrieved from https://apps.who.int/iris/bitstream/handle/10665/43944/9241561009_eng.pdf

Wu, L.-T., Blazer, D. G., Swartz, M. S., Burchett, B., Brady, K. T., & NIDA AAPI Workgroup. (2013). Illicit and nonmedical drug use among Asian Americans, Native Hawaiians/Pacific Islanders, and mixed-race individuals. *Drug and Alcohol Dependence, 133*(2), 360–367. doi:10.1016/j .drugalcdep.2013.06.008

Wu, L.-T., Zhu, H., & Swartz, M. S. (2016). Treatment utilization among persons with opioid use disorder in the United States. *Drug and Alcohol Dependence, 169*, 117–127. doi:10.1016/j .drugalcdep.2016.10.015

Yarnall, K. S. H., Pollak, K. I., Østbye, T., Krause, K. M., & Michener, J. L. (2003). Primary care: Is there enough time for prevention? *American Journal of Public Health, 93*(4), 635–641. doi:10.2105/ajph.93.4.635

CHAPTER 3

Epidemiology of Opioids

KEY TERMS

CDC Guidelines for Prescribing Opioids
Cirrhosis
HIV
HCV
Incidence
Medicare
Mu-opioid Receptor (µOR)
National Survey on Drug Use and
   Health (NSDUH)

Percutaneous (parenteral)
Prevalence
Substance Abuse and Mental
   Health Service Administration
   (SAMHSA)
Syringe Service Program
Tapering
Treatment Episode Data Set
   (TEDS)

LEARNING OBJECTIVES

- Describe the prevalence of opioid use (prescriptions, heroin, fentanyl, etc.)
- Explain risk of infectious disease associated with injection drug use (HIV, HCV)
- Identify the prevalence of opioid use disorders
- Offer explanations for the gap between the number of people who need treatment
  (have an opioid use disorder), the number who seek treatment (treatment
  admissions) and the number who complete treatment.

Chapter 3 addresses where we are in the epidemic. It describes the prevalence of opioid use (prescriptions, heroin, fentanyl, etc.) as well as recent trends in use, availability, and sequela associated with injection drug use (HIV, HCV). It continues with an overview of the prevalence of opioid use disorders, treatment need, treatment admissions and completion.

Recent Opioid Use

The National Survey on Drug Use and Health (NSDUH) provides information on tobacco, alcohol, drug use and mental health in the United States. Results from the 2018 NSDUH suggest that 53.2 million Americans (19.4%) over age 12 used an illicit substance in the past year (Substance Abuse and Mental Health Services Administration, 2019a).

Approximately 10.3 million people aged 12 or older (about 3.7% of the population) in 2018 misused opioids in the past year. Nationally, the percentage of people aged 12 or older in 2018 who were past-year opioid misusers has declined significantly every year since 2015. Although greater detail is provided in the sections that follow, 9.9 million people aged 12 or older in 2018 had misused prescription pain relievers in the past year compared with 808,000 people who used heroin. Most people who misuse prescription pain relievers had misused only prescription pain relievers in the past year—they had not used heroin (9.4 million or 92.1% of the population that misused an opioid). Of the 808,000 people who used heroin, 506,000 people (62.6%) also misused pain relievers in the past year, while just 5.1% of people who misused prescription pain relievers had also used heroin in the past year (Substance Abuse and Mental Health Services Administration, 2019a). We will delve more deeply into the relationship between prescription opioid misuse and heroin use later in this chapter.

Prescription Pain Medication Misuse

In 2018, approximately 19% of Americans who reported any illicit drug use in the last year misused a prescription pain medication (3.6% of the total population). According to the NSDUH definition, prescription drug use without a prescription of one's own or use at a higher dosage or more often than prescribed constitutes misuse. As a nation, the use of illicit prescription pain medication has dropped significantly every year since 2015 when it represented 4.7% of the total population (Substance Abuse and Mental Health Services Administration, 2019a).

The NSDUH captures several categories of prescription pain relievers. These include hydrocodone, oxycodone, tramadol, codeine, morphine, prescription fentanyl, buprenorphine, oxymorphone, hydromorphone, Demerol®, methadone, and any other prescription pain reliever. In 2018, hydrocodone products were the most misused subtype of prescription pain relievers. They include: Vicodin®, Lortab®, Norco®, Zohydro® ER, and generic hydrocodone. Used by 3.4 million (1.2% of the population), oxycodone was the next most frequently misused pain reliever. The family of oxycodone products include OxyContin®, Percocet®, Percodan®, Roxicodone®, and generic oxycodone. Please see **Figure 3-1**.

> "CPD [controlled prescription drugs] abuse continues to be the nation's fastest growing drug problem. Rates of CPD abuse remain high, with individuals abusing CPDs at a higher prevalence rate than any illicit drug except marijuana. Pain relievers are the most common type of CPDs taken illicitly and are the CPDs most commonly involved in overdose incidents." 2013 Drug Threat Assessment Summary, Drug Enforcement Administration (2013)

Fentanyl products have been widely talked about in the popular media. In 2018, there were 269,000 people aged 12 or older who misused prescription fentanyl products, which is about 0.1% of the population. However, this

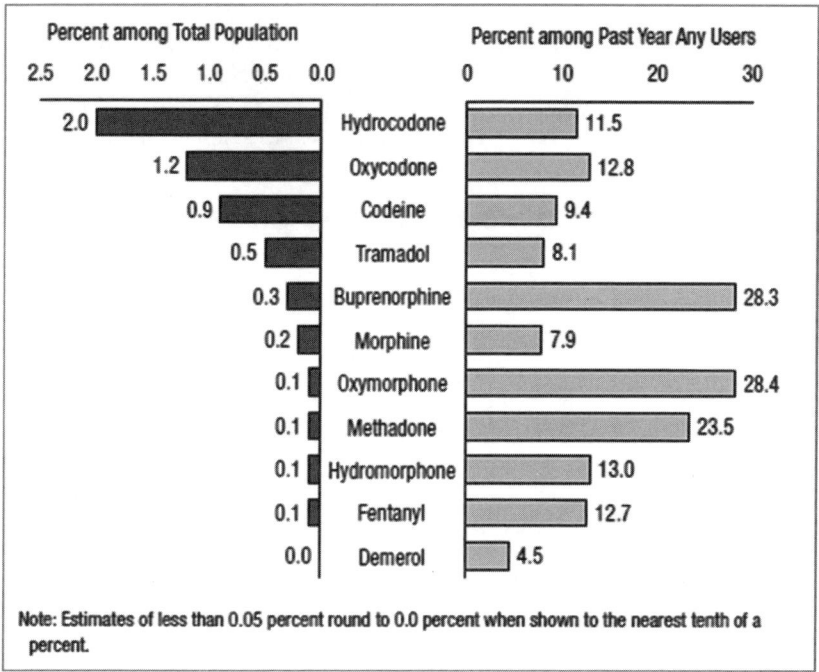

Figure 3-1 Prescription Pain Medication Misuse.

Substance Abuse and Mental Health Services Administration. (2019a). *Key substance use and mental health indicators in the United States: Results from the 2018 National Survey on Drug Use and Health* (HHS Publication No. PEP19-5068, NSDUH Series H-54). Rockville, MD: Author. Retrieved from https://www.samhsa.gov/data/sites/default /files/cbhsq-reports/NSDUHNationalFindingsReport2018/NSDUHNationalFindingsReport2018.pdf

fentanyl misuse estimate likely underrepresents people who misused fentanyl that was illicitly manufactured (Substance Abuse and Mental Health Services Administration, 2019a).

Opioid Medication Misuse?

In 2018, among adolescents aged 12 to 17, 2.8% misused prescription pain relievers, compared with 5.5% of young adults aged 18 to 25 and 3.4% among those aged 26 or older (Substance Abuse and Mental Health Services Administration, 2019a). In the last year, an estimated 5.5 million people aged 12 or older misused these products, corresponding with 2% of the population. NSDUH respondents were asked to report their reasons for misusing the prescription pain reliever the last time they used it. Those who reported more than one reason for misusing the last prescription pain reliever were asked to report the main reason. Among NSDUH participants 12 and older who misused prescription pain relievers in the past year, the most common main reason for their last misuse of a pain reliever was to relieve physical pain (64%). Other reasons included to feel good or to get high (11%) and to relax/relieve tension (9%). Only 3% gave as their top reason that they were "hooked" or needed to have the drug (Substance Abuse and Mental Health Services Administration, 2019a).

When asked about the source of the medication, more than half (51%) of people 12 and older who misused pain relievers in the past year obtained them the previous time from a friend or relative. More than one-third of people who misused pain relievers in the past year (38%) obtained pain relievers the last time through prescription(s) or stole pain relievers from a healthcare provider. Just 6.5% of respondents bought the last pain reliever they misused from a drug dealer or stranger (Substance Abuse and Mental Health Services Administration, 2019a).

Lots and Lots of Opioid Medication Prescriptions

Over the last several decades, medical (and dental) providers have written numerous generous opioid prescriptions. In 2018, 19% of the adult U.S. population filled an opioid prescription, with an average of 3.6 prescriptions per patient (Schieber et al., 2020). It is important to note that prescribers vary markedly in their opioid prescribing practice patterns. In a study of nearly four million patients between 2003 and 2017, the top 1% of providers prescribed between 42% (2005) and 49% (2008) of opioid doses and accounted for between 18% (2004) and 27% (2017) of all opioid prescriptions (Kiang, Humphreys, Cullen, & Basu, 2020). From 2008 to 2018, the percentage of adults who had an opioid prescription filled declined at an average of 3.5% per year. This represents a 31% overall decline, from 27.8% in 2008 to 19.2% in 2018 (Schieber et al., 2020). This decline provides some indication of how plentiful opioid prescriptions had become and raises questions about why so many were "needed" in the first place, a subject that we discussed in Chapter 2 and we will return to shortly. See **Figure 3-2**.

It is important to note that a statistically higher percentage of women filled at least one opioid prescription over the aforementioned study period. Even as prescriptions declined overall, in 2018, women had approximately 1.5 times greater

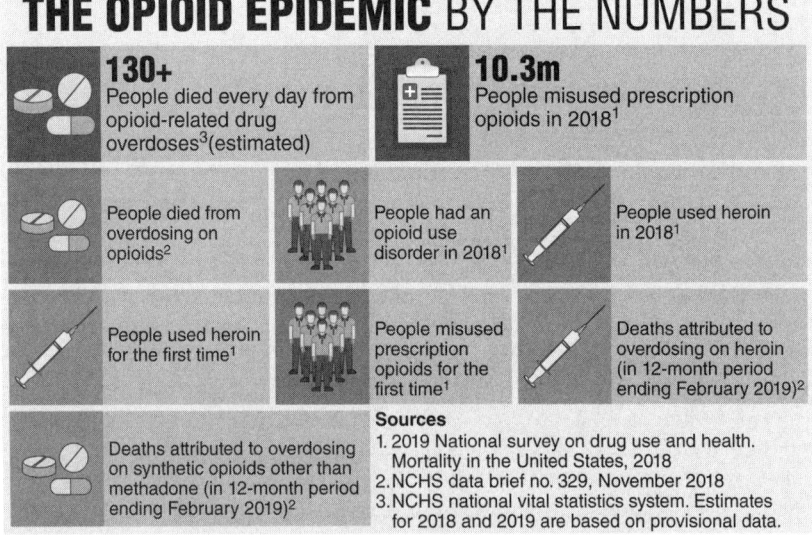

Figure 3-2 The Opioid Epidemic by the Numbers.

odds of filling an opioid prescription than did men (Schieber et al., 2020). The rise in the availability of prescriptions drugs to women was also reflected, in part, in a rapid increase in opioid use disorder diagnosis in hospital delivery wards. In the years from 1999–2014, the national prevalence of opioid use disorder detected at delivery increased by 333%, from 1.5 cases per 1,000 delivery hospitalizations to 6.5, with considerable state variability (Haight, Ko, Tong, Bohm, & Callaghan, 2018).

Prescription rates also differed by age. Compared with people aged 20–24 years (11%), those aged ≥65 years (25%) were approximately 2.6 times as likely to have had an opioid prescription filled in 2018 (Schieber et al., 2020).

Relatively few people who take a prescription opioid develop dependence or an opioid use disorder. However, the chances of developing dependence increase as the duration of the prescription, or the amount of morphine milligram equivalents (MME) increases. For example, in a study of patient medical records spanning the years 2006–2015 among cancer-free patients who received an opioid prescription, approximately 70% of patients had an initial duration of opioids of ≤7 days. Still, seven percent were initially prescribed opioids for ≥31 days. The probability of continued opioid pain reliever use increased among patients when the first prescription supply exceeded 10 days, when a patient received a third prescription, or when the cumulative dose was ≥700 MME (Shah, Hayes, & Martin, 2017).

Opioid Dose Amounts

Between 1999 and 2010, the MME of prescriptions in the United States increased from 180 per capita in 1999 to 782 MME in 2010, followed by a decline to 640 MME per capita by 2015 (Guy et al., 2017). The largest decreases in MMEs occurred from 2010 to 2012, following publication of national guidelines defining high-dose opioid prescribing as >200 MME/day and recommending stronger management strategies (Chou et al., 2009; Management of Opioid Therapy for Chronic Pain Working Group, 2010). The reduction also followed the publication of studies demonstrating a near dose-response relationship with increases in overdose risk as prescribed opioid dosages increased from 20 to 100 MME per day (Bohnert et al., 2011; Dunn et al., 2010; Guy et al., 2017). Please see **Table 3-1**.

Although the MME rate in the United States has fallen since its high (no pun intended) in 2010, it remains higher than many other high-income countries. In 2019, for example, among patients who received a low-risk surgery and who filled a prescription, the mean MME dispensed within 7 days of discharge was highest in the United States at 247 MME versus 169 MME in Canada, and 197 MME in Sweden (Ladha et al., 2019).

Although MMEs per prescription started to drop in 2010, as an apparent offset to the lower MMEs, the average duration of opioid prescriptions increased. Annual prescribing rates for prescriptions of ≥30 days' supply of opioids increased from 17.6 per 100 persons in 2006 to 28.0 per 100 persons in 2012 (an increase of 59%), before leveling off from 2012 to 2015. Annual prescribing rates for prescriptions of <30 days' supply were stable from 2006 to 2012. However, the reduction in number of days appears to be have been partially offset by an increase in MME. The <30 day rate decreased by 20% from 53.2 per 100 persons in 2012 to 42.4 per 100 persons in 2015, but the average days' supply prescribed increased 33.0% from 13.3 in 2006 to 17.7 in 2015 (Guy et al., 2017).

Table 3-1 Percentage of Counties with Changes* in Opioid Prescribing—United States, 2010–2015

Opioid Prescribing Measures	Decrease (%)	Stable (%)	Increase (%)
MME per capita	49.6	27.8	22.6
Overall prescribing rate	46.5	33.8	19.6
High-dose† prescribing rate	86.5	6.7	6.9
Average daily MME per prescription	72.1	25.7	2.2
Average days' supply per prescription	1.1	25.4	73.5

*Among counties with sufficient data, changes of ≥10% were considered to represent an increase or decrease, whereas changes of <10% were considered stable.

†High-dose prescribing rates include prescriptions with daily dosage ≥90 MME.

Guy, G. P., Jr., Zhang, K., Bohm, M. K., Losby, J., Lewis, B., Young, R. . . . Dowell, D. (2017). Vital signs: changes in opioid prescribing in the United States, 2006–2015. *Morbidity and Mortality Weekly Report, 66*(26), 697–704. doi:10.15585/mmwr.mm6626a4

Opioid Use and Location

A discussion of national trends can sometimes imply that the country has had a uniform response to prescription opioids. In fact, the average per capita amounts prescribed in the top-prescribing U.S. counties were approximately six times the amounts prescribed in the lowest-prescribing counties in 2015. As can happen with other medical procedures (Baicker, Buckles, & Chandra, 2006), opioid practice patterns and the systems that supported those patterns varied markedly. Those counties with higher amounts of prescription opioids tended to have more Whites (non-Hispanic), a higher prevalence of diabetes and arthritis, more physicians and dentists, be non-urban, and have higher rates of unemployment and Medicaid enrollment. Counties with the highest prescribing rates were usually rural, White, and poor (Guy et al., 2017). (To compare opioid prescribing rates by county over time, see https://www.cdc.gov/drugoverdose/maps/rxrate-maps.html). Please see **Table 3-2**.

Table 3-2 Sociodemographic Characteristics of Counties by MME Per Capita Quartiles* — United States, 2015

Characteristics	Lowest Quartile	Second Quartile	Third Quartile	Highest Quartile
Population no. (%)	76,225,923 (23.8)	108,825,101 (33.9)	83,254,830 (26.0)	52,330,662 (16.3)
Average MME per capita	202.9	528.5	776.9	1,318.7

Guy, G. P., Jr., Zhang, K., Bohm, M. K., Losby, J., Lewis, B., Young, R. . . . Dowell, D. (2017). Vital signs: changes in opioid prescribing in the United States, 2006–2015. *Morbidity and Mortality Weekly Report, 66*(26), 697–704. doi:10.15585/mmwr.mm6626a4

A description of prescription rates across California may underscore the point. Researchers using California's prescription drug monitoring program extracted prescription records from 2011–2015 (about 30 million people). They aggregated data by zip code areas and found a 300% difference in opioid prescription prevalence by race/ethnicity and income. Their research demonstrates that 44% of adults in the quintile of aggregated zip code areas with the lowest-income but the highest proportion of Whites received at least one opioid prescription each year compared with 16% in the quintile with the highest-income but lowest proportion of Whites. Opioid overdose deaths were concentrated in these lower-income, mostly White regions that received the most prescriptions, such that the poorest/Whitest aggregated zip code areas had an overdose rate that was as much as 10 times greater than the wealthiest aggregated zip code area with the fewest White people (Friedman et al., 2019). Access to prescription medications started to contract across the United States in 2012; however, as recently as 2017, 14 rural counties were among the 15 counties with the highest opioid prescribing rate (García et al., 2019).

Recognizing that in 2012 that healthcare providers wrote 259 million prescriptions for opioid pain medications, enough for every adult in the United States to have a bottle of pills, and that prescribing rates varied across states that could not be explained by the health ailments of the population (Paulozzi, Mack, & Hockenberry, 2014), the CDC eventually issued new guidelines for prescribing opioids (Dowell, Haegerich, & Chou, 2016). The guidelines focused on practitioners' treatment of chronic pain and not pain related to cancer or sickle-cell anemia. The guidelines included a checklist for providers: https://stacks.cdc.gov/view/cdc/38025. By the time the CDC released the report, prescription rates had already been declining, but the release of the report accelerated the reduction in the number of prescriptions and the number of providers prescribing them.

Certainly in the wake but even before the publication of the report, insurance companies were looking for ways to limit access to opioids and began to deny both claims and patients (Demko, 2019). In 2019, the CDC acknowledged that some organizations and providers had used its report to apply strict dosage and duration thresholds without consideration of the needs of particular patients, institute abrupt tapering of drug dosages, and even support sudden opioid discontinuation or dismissal of patients from a physician's practice (Dowell, Haegerich, & Chou, 2019). The CDC clarified the intention of the recommendations and cautioned against hard limits or abrupt tapering (Centers for Disease Control and Prevention, 2019).

Opioid Treatment Medications Used in Ways Other than Intended

Buprenorphine and methadone are prescription medications used to treat patients with opioid use disorders. An estimated 0.3% of the population misused buprenorphine products in the past year, which corresponds to 718,000 people. About 256,000 (0.1%) misused methadone. When one examines the misuse of prescription drug types among patients who report prescription pain reliever subtypes, about 28.3% and 23.5% of past year users of buprenorphine and methadone products misused these products, respectively (Substance Abuse and Mental Health Services Administration, 2019a). Although buprenorphine and morphine misuse represents a small percentage of the total population of misused opioids, the percentages are sufficient to raise diversion concerns among law enforcement authorities, including the Drug Enforcement Agency (Lofwall & Walsh, 2014).

Heroin Use

Among those reporting illicit drug use in the last year, 1.5% used heroin (or .3% of the total population). In 2018, 117,000 people aged 12 or older used heroin for the first time, suggesting that on average approximately 320 people initiated heroin use each day. The percentage of people who had used heroin in the last year had remained at .2% or less between 2002 and 2011, before climbing to .3% in 2012. It has remained there or higher (in 2016, it reached .4%) ever since. In 2018, less than 0.1% of adolescents aged 12 to 17 had used heroin in the past year, compared with .5% among those 18 to 25 in 2018, and .3% of adults aged 26 or older (Substance Abuse and Mental Health Services Administration, 2019a).

Because heroin use rates are relatively low across the population researchers sometimes bundle proximate years together so that estimates will be less susceptible to measurement error. This is the approach that was taken for one NSDUH study that looked at changing heroin trends over time. Results suggest strong increases in heroin use between 2002 and 2017. The annual average rate of past-year heroin use for 2002–2004 was 1.6 per 1,000 and for 2005–2007, 1.8 per 1,000 persons over age 12. From 2011–2013, the rate was 2.6 per 1,000 persons aged ≥12 years. This rate was significantly higher and represents a 62.5% increase since 2002–2004. In addition, the rate of people meeting diagnostic criteria for past-year heroin abuse or dependence increased significantly during the study period, from 1.0 per 1,000 in the years 2002–2004 to 1.9 per 1,000 in the years 2011–2013, which represents a 90.0% increase overall and a 35.7% increase since 2008–2010 (Jones, Logan, Gladden, & Bohm, 2015).

Rates of past-year heroin use were higher among men than women for all time intervals but the gap tightened between 2002–2004 and again from 2011–2013 (Jones et al., 2015). The rates for adolescents (12–17) and those aged 26 and above did not change significantly. However, the rates for those aged 18–25 more than doubled—in 2002–2004, it was 3.5 per 1,000, and by 2011-2013, it was 7.3 per 1,000 (Jones et al., 2015).

Rates of heroin use also changed by racial/ethnic and social class categories. The rate of past-year heroin use among Whites (non-Hispanic) increased by 114.3% from 1.4 per 1,000 in 2002–2004 to 3.0 per 1,000 in 2011–2013. Past-year heroin use increased across household income levels (<$20,000; $20,000–$49,000; ≥$50,000) between 2002–2004 and 2011–2013. Individuals without health insurance as well as those with private or public insurance experienced significant increases in heroin use rates between 2002–2004 and 2011–2013 (Jones et al., 2015).

Most People Who Initiate Heroin Use Do Not Begin De Novo

Most people who use heroin did not start opioid use with heroin. The majority of people who use heroin have a history of nonmedical use of prescription opioid pain relievers. A NSDUH study found that between 2002–2004 and 2008–2010, heroin use increased among people reporting past-year nonmedical use of opioid pain relievers but not among those without nonmedical use. People who use opioids frequently—beyond medical recommendation (i.e., people reporting 100–365 days of nonmedical use) had the highest rate of past-year heroin use and were at increased risk for ever injecting heroin, past-year abuse, or dependence. In 2008–2010, 82.6% of people who frequently used nonmedical pharmaceutical opioids (this is the use of a prescription opioid without or beyond a physician's orders) and who used heroin in the past year reported nonmedical use of opioid pain relievers prior to heroin initiation. In the period between 2002–2004, the percentage was 64% (Jones, 2013). NSDUH data from the last decade (2002–2011) indicate that the rate of heroin initiation among people with a history of nonmedical use of opioid pain relievers was approximately 19 times greater than those with no history of nonmedical use (Muhuri, 2013).

Heroin and Availability

Some have suggested that the increased availability and lower price of heroin in the United States has been a potential contributor to rising rates of heroin use (Jones et al., 2015). The 2013 Drug Threat Assessment Summary, stated that controlled prescription drugs (CPD) were the fastest growing threat (Drug Enforcement Administration, 2013). It is likely that there is a synergistic relationship between the proliferation of pharmaceutical opioids, an increase in the demand for opioids and trends in heroin use.

The DEA noted that the amount of heroin seized at the Southwest border increased significantly between 2008 and 2012 (Drug Enforcement Administration, 2013). Increases in supply can drive down costs (depending on demand), and cheaper goods often increase demand, but most people do not initiate heroin use without first using a prescription opioid. This suggests that the increase in the heroin supply (and lower costs) was meeting a growing demand for opioids at a time when the number of opioid medication prescriptions had started to flatten and then decline.

Heroin Use Over Time

However heroin use is initiated, the population profile of those who use heroin has changed over time. A retrospective mixed-methods study (using quantitative treatment data as well as qualitative interviews) looked back over 50 years of 2,797 patients' data (Cicero, Ellis, Surratt, & Kurtz, 2014). The authors found that it was mostly young men who began using in the 1960s (82.8%; mean age was 16.5 years). They also found that the opioid that those men first used was heroin (80%). As the decades passed, however, the age of those who used heroin increased (mean age, 22.9 years), more women were represented (nearly equal numbers by 2010), and people who used heroin were increasingly suburban and rural (75.2%). Compared with the period when pharmaceutical opioids were not widely available, more of those who were seeking treatment for heroin were first introduced to opioids through prescription drugs such that by the year 2010, about 75% of those seeking treatment for heroin had begun opioid use with an opioid prescription. Whites and people of color were equally represented in those initiating treatment in 1970, but by 2010, nearly 90% of respondents who began heroin use in the last decade were White. Those who initiated heroin use in later decades suggested that the "high" produced by heroin was as important, but they observed that it was often used because it was more accessible and less expensive than prescription opioids (Cicero et al., 2014).

Naloxone Availability

The drug naloxone can reverse an opioid overdose. The CDC recommends that prescribers consider prescribing naloxone with an opioid when: there is a history of overdose or substance use disorder, opioid dosages ≥50 MMEs per day (high-dose), and patients have a concurrent use of benzodiazepines (Dowell, Haegerich, & Chou, 2016). Although the CDC recommends making the drug widely available, in 2018, 236 counties (8.3% of counties with available data) dispensed high-dose opioid prescriptions but did not issue naloxone prescriptions (Guy et al., 2019).

Naloxone has become more available over the last decade. From 2012 to 2018, Naloxone dispensing from retail pharmacies increased from 0.4 per 100,000 in 2012 to 170.2 per 100,000 in 2018. Despite the trend and CDC recommendations, in 2018, only one naloxone prescription was dispensed for every 69 high-dose opioid prescriptions. The highest percentage of dispensed naloxone prescriptions were issued to those with commercial insurance (51%), Medicare (36%), Medicaid (11%), and self-pay (2%). Although insurance coverage can improve affordability, many poor patients with insurance were required to spend money out of pocket, creating another potential barrier to overdose prevention. For example, among prescriptions paid for by Medicare, 71% required out-of-pocket costs; among prescriptions paid for by Medicaid, 44% required out-of-pocket costs; among prescriptions paid for by commercial insurance, 42% required out-of-pocket costs; and 31% of self-pay—those without insurance—had out-of-pocket costs greater than $50.00 (Guy et al., 2019).

Opioids, HIV and Injection Drug Use

In 2015, the National HIV Behavioral Surveillance Survey found a 7% prevalence of HIV infection among persons who inject drugs. Among HIV-negative respondents, 27% reported sharing syringes and 67% reported having vaginal sex without a condom in the last year; only 52% received syringes from a syringe services program and only 34% received all syringes from sterile sources. HIV infection prevalence was higher among Blacks (11%) than Whites (6%). According to the report, more White persons who injected drugs shared syringes (White: 39%; Black: 17%) and injection equipment (White: 61%; Black: 41%) in the past year. The 2015 HIV prevalence rate was lower than the rate in 2012 (11%). The authors note that the change might be explained partially by the sample composition from 2012 to 2015. Between sample years, there was an increase in the percentage of White persons who injected drugs, from 30% in 2012 to 39% in 2015, and White persons who injected drugs in 2012 and 2015 had the lowest HIV prevalence (5% and 6%, respectively) (Burnett, Broz, Spiller, Wejnert, & Paz-Bailey, 2018).

Opioids, HCV, and Injection Drug Use

HCV is transmitted primarily through percutaneous (parenteral) exposure that can result from injection-drug use, needle stick injuries, and inadequate infection control in healthcare settings. Approximately 75–85% of newly infected adults develop a chronic HCV infection. Chronic, untreated HCV infection can lead to hepatic fibrosis, cirrhosis, hepatocellular carcinoma, and liver transplantation and liver-related mortality. Among those chronically infected, approximately 20% will develop cirrhosis within 20 years (Seeff, 2002).

Two decades ago there was disturbing evidence about patients receiving MOUD (methadone); those receiving the recommended dose of 60 mg/d dropped from 80% in 1988 to 36% in 2000, and that programs with greater concentrations of people of color were especially likely to provide low doses (D'Aunno & Pollack, 2002). Since methadone is a long-acting mu-opioid receptor full agonist, patients must be inducted slowly to be sure that the dosage is correct. Receiving lower than the recommended medication dose may not provide sufficient binding to cell receptors, leaving patients with craving or initiating withdrawal, thereby increasing chances of relapse, HIV/HCV infection, and overdose.

Since 2013, new HCV medications have increased the capability of achieving a sustained virologic response (cure) above 90% after 8 to 12 weeks (Centers for Disease Control and Prevention, 2016). The challenge is that HCV incidence increased by 294% nationally from 2010 to 2015 (Centers for Disease Control and Prevention, 2016). The increase is largely attributed to heroin-related injection drug use (Zibbell et al., 2015). Consistent with the findings related to heroin use, follow-up reporting on newly acquired HCV infections reveal that most occur among young White persons who live in non-urban areas (Centers for Disease Control and Prevention, 2016).

Needle-exchange programs have been used to reduce risky injection behaviors and factors that influence virus transmission. Their effectiveness in reducing HIV transmission has been documented in the U.S. and abroad, however evidence for their effectiveness to reduce HCV transmission is less clear (Davis et al., 2017; Hurley et al., 1997). A systematic review of 15 studies lends support to the effectiveness of a broad array of needle-syringe strategies that included structural measures (changes in laws, criminal justice policies, etc.) to reduce both population-level HIV and HCV prevalence (Abdul-Quader et al., 2013).

Emergency Services

During 2006–2010, the percentage of emergency department (ED) visits that had an opioid order prescribed increased among visits involving persons aged 18–44 years (from 34.3% to 39.3%) and 45–64 years (from 33.2% to 38.3%). However, in the next five years, during 2010–2015, the percentage of opioids prescribed decreased among visits for those aged 18–44 years (32.7% in 2015) and 45–64 years (35.2% in 2015). For the decade overall, spanning the years 2006-2015, the percentage remained stable at 21% for 65 years and older (Mundkur et al., 2019).

Growing evidence supports the initiation of buprenorphine induction during emergency department visits for treatment of OUD. The practice is safe, improves treatment retention, and adherence (Cao, Dunham, & Simpson, 2020).

What Is the Prevalence of Opioid Use Disorders (OUD)?

Data from the 2018 National Survey on Drug Use and Health survey indicate that approximately 8.1 million people 12 and older had an illicit drug use disorder in 2018 (Substance Abuse and Mental Health Services Administration,

2019a). Although marijuana use disorder (4.4 million people) was the most common (Substance Abuse and Mental Health Services Administration, 2019a), there were 2,044,469 people (representing 0.7% of the total population) aged 12 and older with an opioid use disorder (OUD). This includes those with prescription pain reliever use disorder (1,355,495 million people), and heroin use disorder (558,406 people) (Substance Abuse and Mental Health Services Administration, 2019a). Opioid use disorders were nearly evenly split between men and women at 52% and 48%, respectively. When broken down by age, 5% of those with an OUD were aged 12–17, 15% of young adults aged 18–25, 23% of adults aged 26–34, 26% of adults aged 35–49, and 30% of adults aged 50 or older (Substance Abuse and Mental Health Services Administration, 2019a).

The 2018 OUD rates by race/ethnicity are consistent with the mortality data reported earlier. Whites had the greatest percentage (67%) followed by rates for other racial groups including Hispanics (17%); Blacks (11%), those self identified as "multiple race" (4%), Asian (1%), Native American/Alaska Natives (0.7%), and Native Hawaiians/Pacific Islanders (0.2%) (Substance Abuse and Mental Health Services Administration, 2019a).

Who Seeks and Completes Opioid Treatment?

The Substance Abuse and Mental Health Services Administration captures treatment data from several sources. One is from the NSDUH, a population survey. The other is from the Treatment Episode Data Set (TEDS), which collects data directly from treatment programs. Both sources help to create an understanding of the demand for and use of treatment for substance use disorders.

The NSDUH survey asks individuals if they have received any treatment, counseling for alcohol or illicit drug use, or had any medical problems associated with alcohol or drug use in the past year (Substance Abuse and Mental Health Services Administration, 2019a). Receiving services at more than one location is recorded. For example, an individual may be admitted to a hospital as an inpatient, or to a specialty care outpatient rehabilitation program, or may receive treatment in primary care (e.g., with buprenorphine), or attend a self-help group. Many individuals use multiple forms of treatment and support such as MOUD and a recovery support group such as Narcotics Anonymous.

The NSDUH estimated that in 2018, 21.2 million people (8 % of the population) aged 12 and older needed treatment over the past year. By contrast, in 2018, 3.7 million people (18% of those who needed treatment) aged 12 and older received any substance use treatment in the past year. The percentage of the population that was in need and actually received treatment has not changed since 2015 (Substance Abuse and Mental Health Services Administration, 2019a).

TEDS data lags a year behind NSDUH information. In 2017, the most recent year for which TEDS data are available, there were 2,005,395 total treatment admissions for people aged 12 and older in the U.S. United States. An individual can be admitted, but that does not mean the person completed treatment. Opioids represented 34% of treatment admissions reported in 2017. Opioid-related treatment admissions are captured in TEDS as either heroin or opiates other than heroin. In 2017, approximately 80% of all opiate-related admissions were for primarily heroin use. Heroin accounted for 27% (533,394 admissions) of total admissions of people aged 12 and older, of whom 63% were male. The average age for primary heroin admissions was 36 years, and non-Hispanic Whites represented 66%, non-Hispanic Blacks accounted for 14%, and Hispanics 13% of people aged 12 and older (Substance Abuse and Mental Health Services Administration, 2019b).

The proportion of treatment admissions for non-heroin opiates increased from 5% in 2007 to 10% from 2011–2012 before it declined to 7% in 2017. There were 148,680 admissions for people aged 12 and older, 53% (78,398) were male and 47% (70,249) were female. The average age of people admitted for non-heroin opioid treatment was 35 years. Non-Hispanic Whites accounted for 79% of admissions, non-Hispanic Blacks 8%, Hispanics 7%, other/multirace 4%, Asian/Pacific Islanders 1%, and American Indian/Alaska Natives 0.1% for people aged 12 and older (Substance Abuse and Mental Health Services Administration, 2019b). Of the primary opioid admissions in 2017 (patients indicate primary drug use upon admission), 41% of heroin admissions and 36% of non-heroin opiate admissions planned to receive MOUD therapy (Substance Abuse and Mental Health Services Administration, 2019b).

In 2017, there were 144,251 people (59,096 women and 85,136 men) aged 12 years and older who were discharged from MOUD therapy. Of those discharged, only 13% completed treatment. Of the remaining discharges 32% transferred, 37% dropped out, 9% terminated treatment, and 9% were discharged from treatment for other reasons (Substance Abuse and Mental Health Services Administration, 2019b). The low treatment completion rates may be some of the lowest of all healthcare services.

Among non-Hispanic Whites discharged from MOUD treatment, only 14% completed treatment. Among those of Hispanic origin, 11% completed treatment and only 9% of non-Hispanic Blacks and 10% of those classified as "other" completed MOUD treatment. Males and females aged 12 years and older completed MOUD at similar rates, 12.5% and 12.8%, respectively (Substance Abuse and Mental Health Services Administration, 2019b).

Data on Access to Medications for Opioid Use Disorders from 2003–2015

Effective treatment for an OUD should include a prescription of FDA-approved medications for withdrawal management, stabilization, and recovery support. Medications include methadone, buprenorphine, and naltrexone. Medications for OUD reduce morbidity and mortality, increase treatment retention, reduce transmission of infectious disease, improve social functioning, and decrease overdose deaths (Volkow, Frieden, Hyde, & Cha, 2014). See **Figure 3-3**.

Although the need for treatment of OUD still often exceeds capacity at the local, state, and national levels, there has been an increase in access to medications for the treatment for OUD. Between 2003 and 2016, the number of opioid treatment programs (OTPs: programs that receive special certification from SAMHSA and the DEA to offer methadone; many also offer buprenorphine) increased from approximately 1,100 to almost 1,500 (Alderks, 2017). The percentage of OTPs offering buprenorphine has also increased from 11% to 58% between 2004 and 2015. In turn, the number of clients receiving buprenorphine at OTPs increased

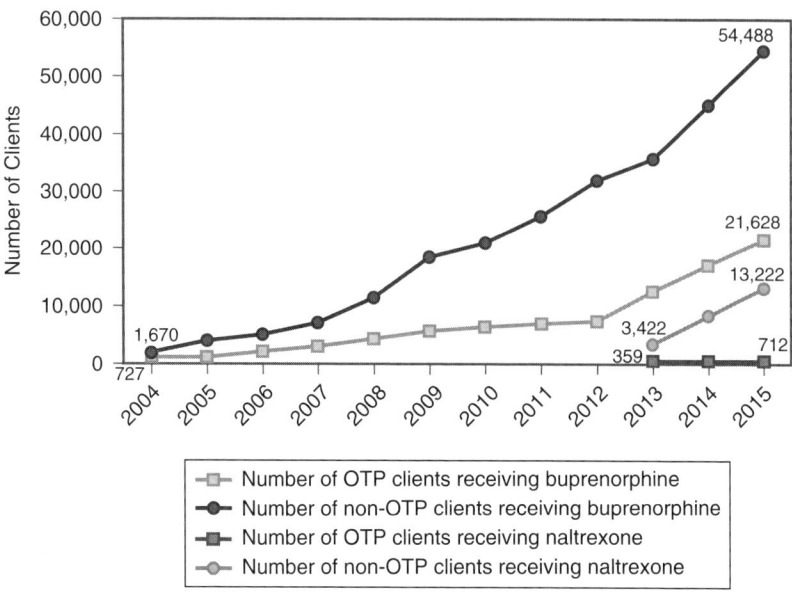

Figure 3-3 Clients Receiving Buprenorphine at OTP and non-OTP 2004-2015.

Alderks, C. E. (2017). Trends in the use of methadone, buprenorphine, and extended-release naltrexone at substance abuse treatment facilities: 2003-2015 (update). *The CBHSQ Report.* Retrieved from https://www.samhsa.gov/data/sites/default/files/report_3192/ShortReport-3192.pdf

from 727 in 2004 to 21,236 in 2015. And the number of clients receiving methadone increased from 227,003 in 2003 to 356,843 in 2015. The percentage of non-OTP facilities prescribing buprenorphine also increased from 5% to 21% between 2004 and 2015, including specialty care substance abuse treatment facilities as well as primary care. These non-OTP programs treated 1,670 clients in 2004 with buprenorphine and that number rose to 54,488 in 2015 (Alderks, 2017). Despite such increases in availability, although treatment for pregnant women is safe, most pregnant women do not receive medication-assisted treatment in spite of rates of OUD having sharply increased among pregnant women (Terplan, Longinaker, & Appel, 2015). Comparing OUD treatment for pregnant women across seven different studies, Lund et al. (2013) found no significant differences in maternal outcomes, neonatal outcomes, or serious adverse outcomes for buprenorphine-naloxone compared with buprenorphine alone, methadone maintenance, or methadone-assisted withdrawal.

Access to extended-release injectable naltrexone (ERIN) increased in both OTPs and non-OTP settings between 2011 and 2015. OTPs offering ERIN increased from 11% in 2011 to 23% in 2015 (from 359 to 712 patients); and non-OTPs increased ERIN access from 8% in 2011 to 16% in 2015 (from 3,422 to 6,323 patients). This does not include ERIN services received through independent medical professionals (Alderks, 2017).

The Accountable Care Act coupled with Medicaid expansion initiated a considerable shift in ownership of substance use disorder treatment centers. Private nonprofit, for-profit, and local, state, federal, or tribal government entities operating SUD treatment facilities shifted significantly between 2008 and 2018. Private nonprofits operating substance-abuse treatment facilities decreased by 6%

between 2008 and 2018 (from 58% to 52% of facilities), while private for-profit facilities increased from 29% to 38% (Substance Abuse and Mental Health Services Administration, 2018b). Treatment center ownership has implications for access, quality, treatment retention and completion (D'Aunno, Friedmann, Chen, & Wilson, 2015; Friedmann, Lemon, Stein, & D'Aunno, 2003).

Discussion Questions

1. What might explain variations in opioid misuse by gender, race, and age?
2. What explains the wide county variations in opioid prescriptions?
3. What is the relationship between opioid prescription potency (as measured by MMEs) and overdoses?
4. Why do people misuse opioid medications?
5. Might there be a relationship between the misuse of opioid medications and heroin use? If yes, what might it be?
6. Why do you think so few people who need treatment for an opioid use disorder receive or complete it?
7. What might explain the low rate of naloxone prescribing relative to opioid prescriptions?

References

Abdul-Quader, A. S., Feelemyer, J., Modi, S., Stein, E. S., Briceno, A., Semaan, S., . . . & Des Jarlais, D. C. (2013). Effectiveness of structural-level needle/syringe programs to reduce HCV and HIV infection among people who inject drugs: a systematic review. *AIDS and Behavior, 17*(9), 2878–2892.

Alderks, C. E. (2017). Trends in the use of methadone, buprenorphine, and extended-release naltrexone at substance abuse treatment facilities: 2003-2015 (update). *The CBHSQ Report*. Retrieved from https://www.samhsa.gov/data/sites/default/files/report_3192/ShortReport-3192.pdf

Baicker, K., Buckles, K. S., & Chandra, A. (2006). Geographic variation in the appropriate use of Cesarean delivery. *Health Affairs, 25*(Suppl. 1), W355–W367. doi:10.1377/hlthaff.25.w355

Bohnert, A. S., Valenstein, M., Bair, M. J., Ganoczy, D., McCarthy, J. F., Ilgen, M. A., & Blow, F. C. (2011). Association between opioid prescribing patterns and opioid overdose-related deaths. *JAMA, 305*(13), 1315–1321.

Burnett, J. C., Broz, D., Spiller, M. W., Wejnert, C., & Paz-Bailey, G. (2018). HIV infection and HIV-associated behaviors among persons who inject drugs—20 cities, United States, 2015. *Morbidity and Mortality Weekly Report, 67*(1), 23.

Cao, S. S., Dunham, S. I., & Simpson, S. A. (2020). Prescribing Buprenorphine for Opioid Use Disorders in the ED: A Review of Best Practices, Barriers, and Future Directions. *Open Access Emergency Medicine: OAEM, 12*, 261.

Centers for Disease Control and Prevention. (2016). Surveillance for viral hepatitis—United States, 2014. Retrieved from https://www.cdc.gov/hepatitis/statistics/2014surveillance/index.htm

Centers for Disease Control and Prevention. (2019). CDC advises against misapplication of the *Guideline for Prescribing Opioids for Chronic Pain* [Press release]. Retrieved from https://www.cdc.gov/media/releases/2019/s0424-advises-misapplication-guideline-prescribing-opioids.html

Chou, R., Fanciullo, G. J., Fine, P. G., Adler, J. A., Ballantyne, J. C., Davies, P., . . . Miaskowski, C. (2009). Clinical guidelines for the use of chronic opioid therapy in chronic noncancer pain. *The Journal of Pain, 10*(2), 113–130.e122. doi:10.1016/j.jpain.2008.10.008

Cicero, T. J., Ellis, M. S., Surratt, H. L., & Kurtz, S. P. (2014). The changing face of heroin use in the United States: A retrospective analysis of the past 50 years. *JAMA Psychiatry, 71*(7), 821–826.

D'Aunno, T., & Pollack, H. A. (2002). Changes in methadone treatment practices: results from a national panel study, 1988-2000. *JAMA, 288*(7), 850–856. doi:10.1001/jama.288.7.850

D'Aunno, T., Friedmann, P. D., Chen, Q., & Wilson, D. M. (2015). Integration of substance abuse treatment organizations into accountable care organizations: Results from a national survey. *Journal of Health Politics, Policy and Law, 40*(4), 797–819.

Davis, S. M., Daily, S., Kristjansson, A. L., Kelley, G. A., Zullig, K., Baus, A., . . . & Fisher, M. (2017). Needle exchange programs for the prevention of hepatitis C virus infection in people who inject drugs: a systematic review with meta-analysis. *Harm reduction journal, 14*(1), 1–15.

Demko, P. (2019, February 12). Health plans don't want patients on opioids. So what are they doing for pain? *Politico.* Retrieved from https://www.politico.com/story/2019/02/12/health-insurance-opioids-pain-1106969

Dowell, D., Haegerich, T. M., & Chou, R. (2016). CDC guideline for prescribing opioids for chronic pain—United States, 2016. *MMWR Recommendations and Reports, 65*(No. RR-1), 1–49. doi:10.15585/mmwr.rr6501e1

Dowell, D., Haegerich, T., & Chou, R. (2019). No Shortcuts to safer opioid prescribing. The *New England Journal of Medicine, 380*(24), 2285–2287. doi:10.1056/NEJMp1904190

Dowell, D., Haegerich, T. M., & Chou, R. (2016). CDC guideline for prescribing opioids for chronic pain—United States, 2016. *JAMA, 315*(15), 1624–1645.

Drug Enforcement Administration Office of Intelligence Warning, Plans and Programs. (2013). *National drug threat assessment summary: 2013.* Washington, DC: U.S. Department of Justice. Retrieved from https://www.dea.gov/sites/default/files/2018-07/DIR-017-13%20NDTA%20Summary%20final.pdf

Dunn, K. M., Saunders, K. W., Rutter, C. M., Banta-Green, C. J., Merrill, J. O., Sullivan, M. D., . . . Psaty, B. M. (2010). Opioid prescriptions for chronic pain and overdose: A cohort study. *Annals of Internal Medicine, 152*(2), 85–92.

Friedman, J., Kim, D., Schneberk, T., Bourgois, P., Shin, M., Celious, A., & Schriger, D. L. (2019). Assessment of racial/ethnic and income disparities in the prescription of opioids and other controlled medications in California. *JAMA Internal Medicine, 179*(4), 469–476.

Friedmann, P. D., Lemon, S. C., Stein, M. D., & D'Aunno, T. A. (2003). Accessibility of addiction treatment: Results from a national survey of outpatient substance abuse treatment organizations. *Health Services Research, 38*(3), 887–903.

García, M. C., Heilig, C. M., Lee, S. H., Faul, M., Guy, G., Iademarco, M. F., . . . Gray, J. (2019). Opioid prescribing rates in nonmetropolitan and metropolitan counties among primary care providers using an electronic health record system—United States, 2014–2017. *Morbidity and Mortality Weekly Report, 68*(2), 25–30. doi:10.15585/mmwr.mm6802a1

Guy, G. P., Jr., Haegerich, T. M., Evans, M. E., Losby, J. L., Young, R., & Jones, C. M. (2019). Vital signs: Pharmacy-based naloxone dispensing—United States, 2012–2018. *Morbidity and Mortality Weekly Report, 68*(31), 679–686. doi:10.15585/mmwr.mm6831e1

Guy, G. P., Jr., Zhang, K., Bohm, M. K., Losby, J., Lewis, B., Young, R., . . . Dowell, D. (2017). Vital signs: Changes in opioid prescribing in the United States, 2006–2015. *MMWR. Morbidity and Mortality Weekly Report, 66*(26), 697–704. doi:10.15585/mmwr.mm6626a4

Haight, S., Ko, J., Tong, V., Bohm, M., & Callaghan, W. (2018). Opioid use disorder documented at delivery hospitalization—United States, 1999–2014. *Morbidity and Mortality Weekly Report, 67,* 845–849. doi:10.15585/mmwr.mm6731a1

Hurley, S. F., Jolley, D. J., & Kaldor, J. M. (1997). Effectiveness of needle-exchange programmes for prevention of HIV infection. *The Lancet, 349*(9068), 1797–1800.

Jones, C. M. (2013). Heroin use and heroin use risk behaviors among nonmedical users of prescription opioid pain relievers–United States, 2002–2004 and 2008–2010. *Drug and Alcohol Dependence, 132*(1-2), 95–100.

Jones, C. M., Logan, J., Gladden, R. M., & Bohm, M. K. (2015). Vital signs: Demographic and substance use trends among heroin users—United States, 2002–2013. *Morbidity and Mortality Weekly Report, 64*(26), 719–725. Retrieved from https://www.cdc.gov/mmwr/preview/mmwrhtml/mm6426a3.htm

Kiang, M. V., Humphreys, K., Cullen, M. R., & Basu, S. (2020). Opioid prescribing patterns among medical providers in the United States, 2003-17: retrospective, observational study. *British Medical Journal, 368*:16968.

Ladha, K. S., Neuman, M. D., Broms, G., Bethell, J., Bateman, B. T., Wijeysundera, D. N., . . . Newcomb, C. W. (2019). Opioid prescribing after surgery in the United States, Canada, and Sweden. *JAMA Network Open, 2*(9), e1910734–e1910734.

Lofwall, M. R., & Walsh, S. L. (2014). A review of buprenorphine diversion and misuse: The current evidence base and experiences from around the world. *Journal of Addiction Medicine, 8*(5), 315.

Lund, I. O., Fischer, G., Welle-Strand, G. K., O'grady, K. E., Debelak, K., Morrone, W. R., & Jones, H. E. (2013). A comparison of buprenorphine + naloxone to buprenorphine and methadone in the treatment of opioid dependence during pregnancy: Maternal and neonatal outcomes. *Substance Abuse: Research and Treatment, 7*, 61–74. doi:10.4137/SART.S10955

Management of Opioid Therapy for Chronic Pain Working Group. (2010). VA/DoD clinical practice guideline for management of opioid therapy for chronic pain.

Muhuri, P. K. G., Joseph C.; Davies, & M. Christine. (2013). Associations of nonmedical pain reliever use and initiation of heroin use in the United States. *CBHSQ Data Review*. Retrieved from https://www.samhsa.gov/data/sites/default/files/DR006/DR006/nonmedical-pain-reliever -use-2013.htm

Mundkur, M. L., Franklin, J. M., Abdia, Y., Huybrechts, K. F., Patorno, E., Gagne, J. J., . . . Bateman, B. T. (2019). Days' supply of initial opioid analgesic prescriptions and additional fills for acute pain conditions treated in the primary care setting—United States, 2014. *Morbidity and Mortality Weekly Report, 68*(6), 140–143. doi:10.15585/mmwr.mm6806a3

Paulozzi, L. J., Mack, K. A., & Hockenberry, J. M. (2014). Vital signs: Variation among States in prescribing of opioid pain relievers and benzodiazepines—United States, 2012. *Morbidity Mortality Weekly Report, 63*(26), 563–568. Retrieved from https://www.cdc.gov/mmwr/preview /mmwrhtml/mm6326a2.htm

Schieber, L., Guy, G. J., Seth, P., & Losby, J. (2020). Variation in adult outpatient opioid prescription dispensing by age and sex—United States, 2008–2018. *Morbidity and Mortality Weekly Report, 69*, 298–302. doi:10.15585/mmwr.mm6911a5

Seeff, L. B. (2002). Natural history of chronic hepatitis C. *Hepatology, 36*(5B), s35–s46.

Shah, A., Hayes, C. J., & Martin, B. C. (2017). Characteristics of initial prescription episodes and likelihood of long-term opioid use—United States, 2006–2015. *Morbidity and Mortality Weekly Report, 66*, 265–269. doi:10.15585/mmwr.mm6610a1

Substance Abuse and Mental Health Services Administration. (2018a). *Data Archive: National Survey on Drug Use and Health*. Retrieved from https://pdas.samhsa.gov/#/survey/NSDUH -2018-DS0001/crosstab/?results_received=false&run_chisq=false&weight=ANALWT_C

Substance Abuse and Mental Health Services Administration. (2018b). *National Survey of Substance Abuse Treatment Services (N-SSATS): Data on Substance Abuse Treatment Facilities*. Retrieved from https://www.samhsa.gov/data/sites/default/files/cbhsq-reports/NSSATS-2018.pdf

Substance Abuse and Mental Health Services Administration. (2019a). *Key substance use and mental health indicators in the United States: Results from the 2018 National Survey on Drug Use and Health* (HHS Publication No. PEP19-5068, NSDUH Series H-54). Rockville, MD: Author. Retrieved from https://www.samhsa.gov/data/sites/default/files/cbhsq-reports/NSDUH NationalFindingsReport2018/NSDUHNationalFindingsReport2018.pdf

Substance Abuse and Mental Health Services Administration. (2019b). *Treatment Episode Data Set (TEDS): 2017. Admissions to and discharges from publicly-funded substance use treatment*. Rockville, MD: Author. Retrieved from https://www.samhsa.gov/data/sites/default/files/cbhsq -reports/TEDS-2017.pdf

Terplan, M., Longinaker, N., & Appel, L. (2015). Women-centered drug treatment services and need in the United States, 2002–2009. *American Journal of Public Health, 105*(11), e50–e54.

Volkow, N. D., Frieden, T. R., Hyde, P. S., & Cha, S. S. (2014). Medication-assisted therapies— tackling the opioid-overdose epidemic. *New England Journal of Medicine, 370*(22), 2063–2066.

Zibbell, J. E., Iqbal, K., Patel, R. C., Suryaprasad, A., Sanders, K. J., Moore-Moravian, L., . . . Holtzman, D. (2015). Increases in hepatitis C virus infection related to injection drug use among persons aged ≤ 30 years—Kentucky, Tennessee, Virginia, and West Virginia, 2006– 2012. *Morbidity and Mortality Weekly Report, 64*(17), 453–458. Retrieved from https://www.cdc .gov/mmwr/preview/mmwrhtml/mm6417a2.htm

CHAPTER 4

Public Policy and the Epidemic

KEY TERMS

Federal Agencies
National Association of County and City
    Health Officials (NACCHO)
National Association of State Substance
    Abuse and Drug Abuse Directors
    (NASADAD)
Opioids Policy

Policy Context
Policy Research
Politics and Policy
Role of Health Systems
State Level Policy
Syndemic

LEARNING OBJECTIVES

- To gain a better understanding of the policy context in the United States
- To identify key agencies involved in opioid policy
- To acquire knowledge of the systems perspective in opioid epidemic mitigation
- To better understand policy dynamics

Chapter Summary

This chapter provides an overview of goals for a comprehensive substance use disorder treatment system and public policy as it pertains to the opioid epidemic and more specifically Opioid Use Disorders (OUD). Opioid policy in the United States is described within its context of federalism involving federal, state, and local governments, as well as interest groups and other stakeholders. Additionally, key agencies are identified as well as recent legislation; and several policy research and policy advocacy organizations are discussed.

Opioid Policy Landscape

The opioid epidemic, with its various co-occurring conditions, requires a comprehensive systems-based policy response to address its devastating effects and prevent further amplification in the society. As stated by the National Academy of

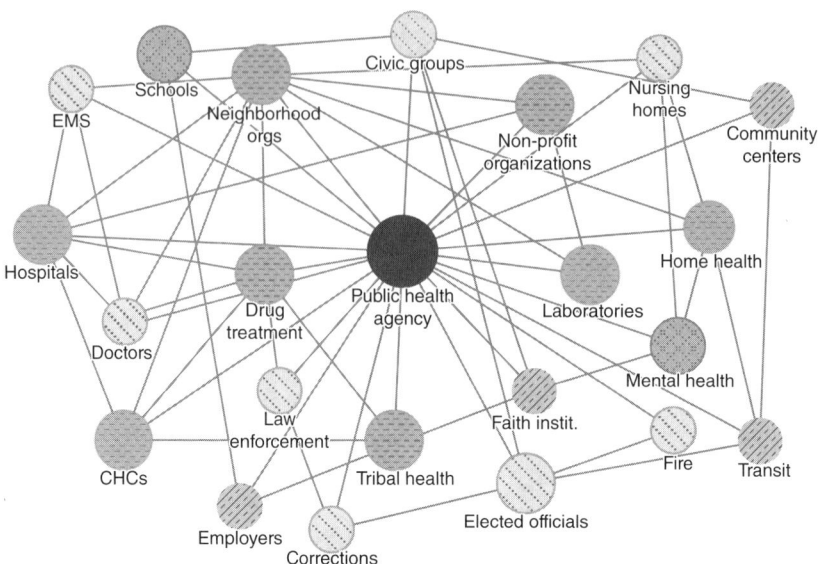

Figure 4-1 Public Health Agency Interconnections.

Reproduced from Centers for Disease Control and Prevention. (n.d.) 10 essential public health services. Retrieved from https://www.cdc.gov/publichealthgateway
/publichealthservices/essentialhealthservices.html

Medicine President Victor J. Dzau, "The complexity of this crisis requires sustained commitment from all stakeholders: health systems, federal and state governments, community organizations, provider groups, payers, industry, nonprofits, and academia. Reversing the opioid epidemic requires a multi-sectoral response—no organization, agency, or sector can solve this problem on their own" (as cited in National Academies of Sciences, Engineering, and Medicine, 2019). As described by Johnson and Davey (2021), there is a web of interconnections between and interdependencies among myriad agencies and organizations working to assure the public's health. This complex system of care can be somewhat visualized in **Figure 4-1**.

Overview of Health Systems

As with HIV/AIDS and COVID-19 epidemic, health systems, including hospitals and community health centers, are in a unique position to increase access to essential services, assure quality of care and patient safety, provide a credentialed professional workforce, and best utilize health information technology, including telemedicine (Johnson, 2018).

The World Health Organization (WHO) defines a healthcare system as (1) all the activities whose primary purpose is to promote, restore, and/or maintain health, and (2) the people, institutions, and resources arranged together to do so. Healthcare systems provide a wide range of clinical services, from primary through subspecialty care. (WHO, 2020). In their multi-year study of health systems around the world, Johnson, Stoskopf, and Shi (2018) found that high performing systems, as measured by quality, access, and cost indicators, incorporated the WHO's essential building blocks as critical success factors. The core components are (i) service delivery; (ii) health workforce; (iii) health information systems; (iv) access to essential

Table 4-1 Health Systems Building Blocks (Critical Success Factors for OUD Treatment)

Service Delivery	Essential Medicines
Essential services for OUD care provided throughout the treatment spectrum from ED, medically managed detoxification, stabilization, inpatient care, recovery, and long-term outpatient services, including behavioral therapy and MOUD.	Medicines used to treat OUD (e.g. methadone and buprenorphine) and to prevent relapse, including Naloxone for use at home and the workplace to reverse overdose.
Health Workforce	**Financial Resources**
A highly skilled professional workforce trained in OUD care, including, typically, OUD-trained physicians and other clinicians, nurses, social workers and counselors, and recovery support personnel.	Adequate funds for prevention, treatment and health promotion that ensure people can use needed services regardless of ability to pay, and provide incentives for providers and users to be efficient.
Health Information and Technology	**Leadership and Governance**
Health information system that includes electronic health records (EHRs), integration with state Prescription Drug Monitoring Programs (PDMPs) and other relevant databases such as CDC, NIDA, Centers for Medicare and Medicaid Services (CMS), and, where appropriate, telemedicine capacity or other "hub and spoke" arrangements.	Hospital-led community-based strategic planning combined with effective oversight, coalition building, regulation, attention to system design, and accountability, including hospital board education and support.

medicines; (v) financing; and (vi) leadership/governance. Each of the six building blocks must be put into place in a manner that assures access and quality. These are shown in **Table 4-1**, as they pertain to OUD care and the inter-relationships between health professionals, federal and state policymakers, and communities.

Goals of a Comprehensive Substance Use Disorder Treatment System

The Pew Charitable Trust lays out four characteristics of an effective substance use disorder treatment system. They have been adapted and appear below.

- Timely: A timely system ensures a continuum of services across ASAM's levels of care that are geographically distributed according to need. The concept of timely should include access to on-demand treatment, or at a minimum, timing of treatment that is consistent with disease severity.
- Comprehensive: Services include screening, diagnosis, withdrawal management, treatment, maintenance, and recovery—across public (e.g. Medicaid/Medicare)

and private insurers. A comprehensive treatment system addresses evidence-based treatment needs for young people, juveniles, pregnant women, and justice-involved persons; it coordinates care between SUDs, mental health, and physical health.

- Evidence-based: Includes financial coverage and utilization of: 1) all FDA-approved medications for the treatment of SUD as well as 2) recommended behavioral health interventions. Evidence-based includes screening and treatment of co-occurring mental health disorders and infectious diseases.
- Sustainable: Optimizes federal funding resources, develops the workforce, maximizes treatment initiation opportunities, focuses on retention, and collaborates with community-based partners to augment treatment services. (The Pew Charitable Trust, 2019)

Substance use disorder treatment, like other forms of treatment, must be paid for. Although every state offers some form of publicly funded SUD treatment, having health insurance increases the chances of gaining access and completing treatment (Abraham et al. 2017). States that expanded Medicaid eligibility under the Affordable Care Act saw a robust increase in SUD treatment admissions in the four years after Medicaid expansion, with 36% more people entering treatment in the 4th year after the state expanded access compared with nonexpansion states. Admissions were greatest for people entering intensive outpatient programs and those seeking MOUD (Saloner and Maclean, 2020).

Even with health insurance, the substance use disorder treatment system, like the disorder, can be complicated. Some of the system was described at the end of Chapter 2 under "Treatment for Opioid Use Disorders" and again at the end of Chapter 3 in the "Who Seeks and Completes Opioid Treatment?" and the "Data on Access to Medications for Opioid Use Disorders from 2003–2015" sections. However, an overview is warranted.

The recent United States Preventive Services Task Force recommendation to support the screening for drug misuse in primary care (USPSTF, 2020) supports an integrated care approach for SUD treatment as described in Chapter 2. Taking primary care as a starting point (but not the only entry point), a healthcare professional may ask a patient about recent drug use employing a validated screening instrument. There are several validated screening instruments for drug use (e.g., NMASSIST (NIDA, 2021) or CAGE-AID (National HIV Curriculum, 2021)).

If a patient indicates recent drug use, the provider will continue to investigate through a brief assessment process. If the brief assessment suggests a problem, the provider will complete a more in-depth assessment to determine diagnosis (using either ICD-10 or DSM-V diagnostic criteria discussed in Chapter 1). There has been no proven efficacy (proof that even under ideal conditions, it is successful) in delivering a brief intervention to reduce opioid use in primary care (Saitz, 2014). Through conversation; however, the medical provider can initiate MOUD treatment (buprenorphine) with the patient's consent. Initiating treatment in the same visit is often preferred since referrals to specialty care treatment are often not completed (Blevins et al. 2018). MOUD should be accompanied by professional behavioral health treatment, peer support, and/or other supports as appropriate for the patient's needs. **Figure 4-2** offers a four-quadrant model that attempts to link disorder severity with treatment setting (CSAT, 2005).

Several population surveys have found that about 50% of those who experience a mental illness during their lives will also experience a substance use disorder

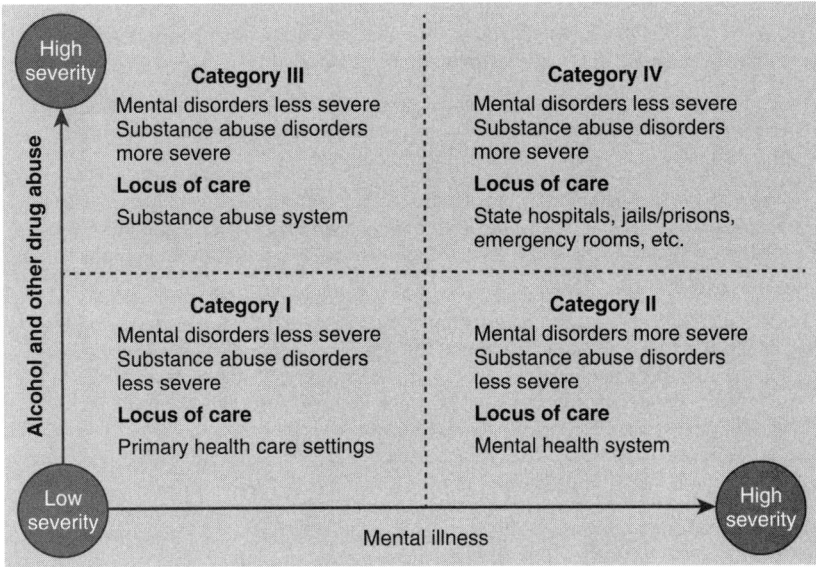

Figure 4-2 Level of Care Quadrants.

Reproduced from Center for Substance Abuse Treatment. (2005). *Substance abuse treatment for persons with co-occurring disorders* (Treatment Improvement Protocol (TIP) Series, No. 42). Retrieved from https://www.ncbi.nlm.nih.gov/books/NBK64184/figure/A74172

(Kelly and Daley, 2013). One study suggests that 43% of people in SUD treatment for misuse of prescription painkillers have a diagnosis or symptoms of mental health disorders, depression and anxiety in particular (Goldner et al., 2014). The recommended levels of care in the four-quadrant model are described in **Figure 4-3**.

Primary care is not the only "door" that patients can use to initiate treatment. As with many other diseases where access is not readily available, people with OUD may go to the hospital emergency room for care. Emergency departments (ED) are federally mandated, under the Emergency Medical Treatment and Active Labor Act (EMTALA) to care for all patients regardless of insurance status and ability to pay. This has led to hospitals receiving a pronounced, direct impact of the epidemic. The overdose ED visit rate quadrupled from 1993 to 2010 (Hasegawa et al., 2014). The EDs located in hospitals are always open and provide access to life-saving medical professionals. A 2018 article in the *New England Journal of Medicine* makes the point as follows:

> For patients who present with opioid overdose, an ED visit represents a critical, time-sensitive point at which initiating lifesaving treatment is possible. Furthermore, EDs are the only venues that are federally mandated, under the Emergency Medical Treatment and Active Labor Act (EMTALA), to care for all patients regardless of their insurance status and ability to pay. Therefore, they serve a segment of the population that is disproportionately vulnerable and disenfranchised, including people who might not be able to receive treatment elsewhere. We believe that striving to deliver evidence-based treatment consistently and effectively for OUD—by thinking of the ED as an integral part of the response to the opioid crisis and the health care system as a whole—could help change the trajectory of the epidemic. (D'Onofrio et al., 2018)

Quadrant I: Low-severity individuals can be accommodated in intermediate outpatient mental health, SUD treatment, or primary care.

Quadrant II: This quadrant includes individuals with high-severity mental disorders who are usually identified as priority clients within the mental health system and who also have low-severity substance use disorders.

Quadrant III: This quadrant includes individuals who have severe substance use disorders and low- or moderate-severity mental disorders. They are generally well accommodated in intermediate-level substance use disorder treatment programs.

Quadrant IV: Quadrant IV is divided into two subgroups. One subgroup includes individuals with serious and persistent mental illness (SPMI) who also have severe and unstable substance use disorders. The other includes individuals with severe and unstable substance use disorders and severe and unstable behavioral health problems. Both groups require intensive, comprehensive, and integrated services for both their substance use and mental disorders.

Figure 4-3 Level of Care.

Data from Center for Substance Abuse Treatment. (2005). *Substance abuse treatment for persons with co-occurring disorders* (Treatment Improvement Protocol (TIP) Series, No. 42). https://www.ncbi.nlm.nih.gov/books/NBK64184/figure/A74172/

Treatment may also be initiated directly through the specialty care system (including outpatient, intensive outpatient, and residential services, corresponding to levels of care outlined by the American Society of Addiction Medicine (https://www.asam.org/asam-criteria/about). SAMHSA offers a treatment locator on its website: https://findtreatment.samhsa.gov/

In addition, treatment may be accessed through the criminal justice system. In a study using treatment admission data from SAMHSA for federally funded substance use treatment facilities in all 50 states, the District of Columbia, and Puerto Rico, 24% were referred to treatment through the criminal justice system in 2014. Of the criminal justice-referred patients, only 4.6% of clients received agonist treatment, compared with 40.9% of those referred by other sources. (Krawczyk et al. 2017).

Economic Policy Challenges

The opioid epidemic cost the U.S. economy more than $1 trillion from 2001 to 2017 (Altarum, 2018). During this period, the annual economic burden of the opioid epidemic surged from $29.1 billion in 2001 to an estimated $115 billion in 2017. The epidemic will likely have cost the nation an additional $500 billion by the end of 2020, according to an analysis by the non profit healthcare research organization Altarum (2018). The greatest cost was associated with lost earnings and productivity from overdose deaths (Ruhm, 2017).

Federal Legislative Policy

For an overview of the U.S. political system, see **Exhibit 4-1**. This will help the reader better understand the political context of federal policy.

EXHIBIT 4-1 Overview of U.S. Political System

As described in the Johnson and Davey (2021) book *Essential of Managing Public Health Organizations*, the federal government has three branches: **legislative** (the Senate and House of Representatives), **executive** (the President and cabinet departments), and **judicial** (federal courts and the U.S. Supreme Court). Each of the states also has its own constitution and its own legislative, executive (governor and cabinet), and judicial branches.

In general, the states can do anything that is not prohibited by the U.S. Constitution or that is contrary to federal policy. A state might choose to embrace its own laws that don't align with federal policy; an example of this would be the regulation of recreational and medical marijuana. The major reserved powers of the state include the authority to regulate commerce within the state and to exercise law enforcement powers. States have the right to pass and enforce laws that promote health, safety, welfare, and "morality." For example, in health promotion, there may be laws pertaining to the use of tobacco products. Elected politicians representing their constituents make decisions and take actions that are broadly referred to as **public policy**. Policies can take the form of new laws; repeals of existing laws; and interpretations and implementations of laws, executive orders, and court rulings. Throughout the policymaking process, the system of constitutional checks and balances prevails. The President (or governor) often plays an important leadership role in key policy issues. The Constitution grants Congress the power to make laws. The legislative process is often cumbersome, as a bill (before it becomes law) goes through both houses of Congress and various committees and subcommittees. Numerous organizations called interest groups, which represent common objectives of their members, try to influence policymakers to protect their members' interests. One example of a powerful interest group is the American Medical Association (AMA). If the President signs the approved bill, it becomes law. The President t also has the power to veto (overturn) a bill passed by Congress. Unless a Presidential veto is overruled by a two-thirds majority of Congress, it fails to become law. Even after a law has been passed, policymaking continues in the form of interpretation and implementation by the federal agency responsible for implementing the law. For example, the Department of Health and Human Services (DHHS) oversees more than 300 programs related to health and welfare services. It is responsible for 12 different agencies that deal with diverse areas related to public health, such as approval of new drugs and medical devices, health science research, services for children and the elderly, and substance abuse.

A recent example of opioids legislation is the Substance Use-Disorder Prevention that Promotes Opioid Recovery and Treatment for Patients and Communities Act, also known as the "SUPPORT Act" of 2019. The legislation makes a variety of legal and regulatory modifications to make OUD treatment more accessible. The law affects every sector of health care, from family medical practices to hospitals to health insurance companies. Perhaps the most significant impact of the legislation is that it removes restrictions for Medicare and Medicaid patients in need of OUD treatment and aims to stop the overprescribing of opioid medications. Key provisions of the act are summarized in **Exhibit 4-2**.

Exhibit 4-2 SUPPORT Act Summary

Overall, the Act aims to facilitate the discovery of alternative non-addictive pain medications, educate the public and clinicians about opioid misuse and help individuals gain access to opioid use disorder treatment. Lastly, the Act strives to reduce the number of opioids circulating in the population.

Medicaid Provisions
The Act temporarily requires coverage of medication for opioid use disorders (MOUD) for patients with Medicaid]. Healthcare providers must check a Medicaid enrollee's prescription history in the prescription drug monitoring program (PDMP) before prescribing controlled substances

Medicare Provisions
Certified opioid treatment programs are now covered for patients with Medicare. Medicare enrollees must undergo an initial examination, which includes screening for an opioid use disorder. The Centers for Medicare and Medicaid Services (CMS) must provide educational resources to Medicare beneficiaries regarding opioid use, pain management, and opioid alternatives. The Act exempts substance-use disorder telehealth services from certain Medicare requirements.

Treatment Provisions
The Act creates a loan repayment program for individuals who work in substance use treatment programs in shortage areas or where drug overdose deaths are high. The Act requires the Substance Abuse and Mental Health Services Administration (SAMHSA) to award grants to create or operate at least 10 opioid recovery centers across the country. The Act increases the number of patients clinicians may treat using MOUD.

Other Provisions
The Act requires that CMS must establish a secure online portal to allow data sharing and prevent or investigate fraud, waste, or abuse.
    Additional funding is provided to the NIH for health sciences research on addiction.

As described by the Commonwealth Fund, "the law is an important step forward, offering a range of policies to prevent new addictions and to expand access to treatment, including MOUD. The law seeks to promote harm-reduction strategies, such as greater distribution of nalaoxone, to reduce deaths. It also authorizes pilot and demonstration projects for states to experiment with ways to expand health provider capacity. However, the law is also notable for what it does *not* include, most prominently, a major, sustained infusion of new funding to expand community-based care for substance use disorders" (Commonwealth Fund, 2020). Unfortunately, the law does not pay for a wide and sustained expansion of SUD treatment, which is desperately needed. In fact, the law does not provide a significant increase in spending for the opioid epidemic at all. The SUPPORT Act is far from what the United States undertook for the HIV/AIDS epidemic, when it enacted sweeping programs like the Ryan White Act and the President's Emergency Plan for AIDS Relief (PEPFAR) to provide the financial resources to fight HIV/AIDS. Furthermore, the SUPPORT Act will likely seem anemic when compared with funding for COVID-19 patient care and epidemic mitigation.

Federal Agency Roles

There are many federal agencies involved in the national effort to mitigate the opioids epidemic. Each agency with its own organizational culture, mission, and political context approaches its efforts somewhat differently. The ideal with a complex epidemic would be to have extensive inter-agency collaboration. The agencies described below work with others at all levels of government: federal, state, and local (see **Exhibit 4-3**).

Exhibit 4-3 **Perspective on Opioid Policies in Other Countries**

As the US continues to develop strategies to fight the opioid epidemic, some countries have already found strategies to avert or combat the crisis. Just like the United States, some other countries are also struggling to tackle their opioid crisis. Below are some countries and what they have done in the last two years regarding the development of policies to regulate opioid use.

Canada
On January 31, 2020.
 Canada and the United States agreed to work more closely together to find solutions to abate the opioid crisis by developing a joint action plan. The two countries will boost their collaboration to combat opioid trafficking, including fentanyl and other synthetic opioids, and address the health consequences of problematic opioid use through public health, law enforcement, and border security cooperation as well as share information and best practices. The United States and Canada have been working together to determine key areas of focus requiring additional cooperation.
 August 26, 2020 - Peterborough, Ontario - Health Canada
 The COVID-19 outbreak has worsened the situation for many Canadians struggling with substance use. Minister for Women and Gender Equality and Rural Economic Development announced more than $1.9 million in funding over the next three years to the Peterborough Police Service. Through this funding, people who use drugs and experience mental health issues will be connected to newly created community-based outreach and support services.
 As part of this project, the Peterborough Police Service is working with local partners to create a community-based outreach team to increase the capacity for front-line community services to help people at risk who are referred by police.

Australia
From January 1, 2020, mandates for smaller pack sizes for opioids, better labeling, warnings and consumer information for opioid pharmaceuticals, and restrictions on the use of fentanyl patches went into effect.

(continues)

Exhibit 4-3 **Perspective on Opioid Policies in Other Countries** *(continued)*

Opioid prescriptions are now available only in smaller quantities without refills for the treatment of non-chronic pain. To be eligible for treatment with opioids, patients will need to be unresponsive or intolerant, or have achieved inadequate relief of their acute pain, to maximum tolerated doses of non-opioid treatments. For chronic pain, increased quantities and/or repeats may be authorized by Services Australia, where the patient meets the restriction requirements.

To be eligible for treatment with high-strength opioids, such as morphine and fentanyl, patients will need to be unresponsive or intolerant, or have achieved inadequate relief of their acute pain, following maximum tolerated doses of other lower-strength opioid treatments.

United Kingdom

The Public Health England report revealed that more than half a million people have been on opioids for more than three years.

In short, Britain is in danger of replicating the US opioid crisis. Doctors in the UK get to spend very little time with their patients compared with other European countries. Trying to find viable alternatives to painkillers for chronic pains for patients in a 10-minute session is a challenge. Leading SUD treatment experts at UK Addiction Treatment Centers (UKAT) has seen a 33% increase in the number of patients being treated for opioid prescription drug SUD in the last two years.

Portugal

Portugal became the first country to decriminalize all drugs. Drugs were still illegal, and people would still be prosecuted for supplying or trafficking drugs, but those caught with small quantities would not be arrested.

Decriminalization was the most prominent part of a package of reforms designed to take a humane approach to SUD, to treat it as a disease rather than a moral failing. Drug users would be viewed as patients, not as criminals, and they would be met with treatment, rather than incarceration.

The approach has demonstrated promise. Over the last nearly two decades, the number of heroin users in Portugal has been cut by two-thirds and drug-related deaths have plummeted from more than one a day in 1999 to 30 in all of 2016. The decrease in new drug-related HIV infections has been even more striking, with 18 recorded in 2016, according to a 2019 report by the European Monitoring Centre for Drugs and Drug Addiction, compared with 907 in 2000.

In 2017, the Portuguese opened supervised drug consumption facilities, building upon mobile outreach methods. Here, health professionals provide a safe, hygienic space to consume drugs and can rapidly intervene in case of complications or overdose.

Germany

Germany is following the European tendency of minimizing the harmful effects that opioids inflict on society.

The German healthcare system is primarily state funded, with only a minority of its costs covered by private insurance. Consequently, German doctors are less susceptible to pressure from Big Pharma to write unnecessary opioid prescriptions, a major contributing factor to the opioid crisis in the United States.

The German healthcare system tends to utilize "harm reduction" strategies that the Organization for Economic Cooperation and Development have classified as "best practices" in response to OUD. Germans with OUD are better able than Americans to safely use opioids in supervised drug consumption centers and benefit from needle/syringe exchanges.

Opioid prescription in Germany is tightly regulated by the Narcotic Drugs Prescription Ordinance and by the German Narcotic Drugs Act, which entered into force in 1992.

The BtMVV gives detailed information on prescription rules (maximum quantities of opioids prescribed within a timeframe, maximum amount of different opioids prescribed at once). In Germany, all opioids must be prescribed by a medical doctor, a veterinarian, or a dentist. All opioids—except Tramadol and Codeine (normal prescription only)—require special narcotic prescriptions known as "BtM"-prescriptions.

Germany is the second largest consumer of opioid pain relievers in Europe behind the United Kingdom and ahead of Spain. However, even though patterns of opioid prescription follow similar trends than other developed countries, there are no signs of an opioid epidemic in Germany so far. Studies could currently not find a need for urgent health policy interventions regarding opioid prescription practices in Germany.

References

Goverment of Canada. (2018). Enforcement: Canadian drugs and substances strategy. Retrieved from https://www.canada.ca/en/health-canada/services /substance-use/canadian-drugs-substances-strategy/enforcement.html

Walsh, J. (2020). The opioid crisis in Australia. Retrieved from https://www .dwfoxtucker.com.au/2020/02/the-opioid-crisis-in-australia/

Faria, L. M. (2019). Portugal solved it drug crisis. Why can't America do the same? *HuffPost*. Retrieved from https://www.huffpost.com/entry/portugal -america-drug-crisis-decriminalize_n_5dbad944e4b066da552d4a6d

Werber, A., Marschall, U., L'hoest, H., Hauser, W., Moradi, B., & Schiltenwolf, M. (2015). Opioid therapy in the treatment of chronic pain conditions in Germany. *Pain Physician, 18*(3), E323–E331. https://pubmed.ncbi.nlm.nih.gov/26000679/

Contributed by Iboro Udoete, MD.

Health Resources and Services Administration (HRSA)

- In September 2018, HRSA awarded $352 million in new funding to expand access to substance use disorder and mental health services Federally Qualified Health Centers (FQHCs) across the nation. FQHCs are community-based health centers that provide primary care services in underserved areas. They must provide care on a sliding fee scale based on ability to pay and operate under a governing board that includes patients. FQHCs integrate access to pharmacy, mental health, SUD, and oral health services in areas with limited access to affordable health care services.
- They initiated the Integrated Behavioral Health Services (IBHS) funding, which will help health centers increase access to high-quality, integrated mental health and substance use disorders (SUD) services, including OUD.

Substance use disorder prevention services provide safe and effective pain management, and implement MOUD as part of integrated behavioral health-care services (HRSA, n.d.-a, n.d.-b).

Indian Health Services (IHS)

- The IHS supports safe and effective therapies to help patients and providers best manage pain and opioid use disorder. The IHS is working to eliminate stigma and encourage positive patient outcomes through appropriate and effective pain management, reducing overdose deaths from heroin and prescription opioid misuse, and improve access to culturally appropriate treatment. The IHS coordinates, collaborates, and participates in listening sessions, formal consultations, and community roundtables to ensure Heroin Opioid and Pain Efforts (HOPE) committee work is relevant to tribal communities.
- In addition, the HOPE committee strives to expand availability of co-prescribed and first-responder access to naloxone for patients at risk for opioid overdose, to expand Neonatal Opioid Withdrawal Syndrome (NOWS)/Neonatal Abstinence Syndrome (NAS) guidelines to increase screening and referral to treatment for pregnant and parenting mothers, and to improve data collection, analysis, and evaluation to target strategies to impact pain management and addiction in tribal populations.
- IHS has adopted the HHS 5-Point Strategy to Combat the Opioid Crisis. In order to put evidence-based opioid prescribing strategies into practice, IHS supports increasing the capacity of health-care providers and systems of care. Regional (and if indicated, national) care teams should share information, since effective local and national opioid stewardship requires ongoing review and study of available chronic pain management innovations (IHS, n.d.).

Centers for Disease Control and Prevention (CDC)

- Overdose Data to Action (OD2A) is a 3-year cooperative agreement through which CDC funds health departments in 47 states, Washington DC, two territories, and 16 cities and counties for surveillance and prevention efforts. These efforts include timelier tracking of nonfatal and fatal drug overdoses, improving toxicology to better track polysubstance-involved deaths, enhancing linkage to care for people with OUD and risk for opioid overdose, improving prescription drug monitoring programs, implementing health systems interventions, partnering with public safety, and implementing other innovative surveillance and prevention activities.
- The CDC developed and published the *CDC Guideline for Prescribing Opioids for Chronic Pain* to provide recommendations for the prescribing of opioid pain medication for patients 18 and older in primary care settings (Dowell et al., 2016).
- The CDC awarded $155 million to states to fight the opioid epidemic and has distributed an additional $27 million to nine organizations to help support staffing and training. The CDC has several goals to prevent opioid-related deaths, including increasing public awareness about the risks (CDC, n.d.).

National Institutes of Health (NIH)

- The NIH, a component of HHS, is the nation's leading medical research agency helping to solve the opioid crisis by discovering new and better ways to prevent opioid misuse, treat OUD, and manage pain.
- In April 2018 at the National Prescription Drug Abuse and Heroin Summit, NIH announced the launch of the HEAL (Helping to End Addiction Long-term) Initiative, an aggressive, trans-agency effort to speed scientific solutions to stem the national opioid public health crisis.
- There are also specialized institutes and agencies under the NIH umbrella. The most prominent as it pertains to substance abuse and misuse is the National Institute of Drug Abuse (NIDA), a research institute whose mission is to advance science on the causes and consequences of drug use and addiction and to apply that knowledge to improve individual and public health (NIDA, 2020; NIH, 2021).

U.S. Food and Drug Administration (FDA)

- The FDA began to focus on four priority areas in 2018: Reduce the burden of addiction crises that are threatening American families; leverage innovation and competition to improve health care, broaden access, and advance public health goals; empower consumers to make better and more informed decisions about their diets and health; and expand the opportunities to use nutrition to reduce morbidity and mortality from disease and strengthen the FDA's scientific workforce and its tools for efficient risk management.
- On October 24, 2018, the President signed into law the SUPPORT for Patients and Communities Act. Under section 3002, the Commissioner of Food and Drugs is required to develop evidence-based opioid analgesic prescribing guidelines for indication-specific treatment of acute pain for the relevant therapeutic areas where such guidelines do not exist.
- FDA's Opioid Analgesic Risk Evaluation and Mitigation Strategy (REMS), approved on September 18, 2018, is one strategy among multiple national and state efforts to reduce the risk of abuse, misuse, OUD, overdose, and deaths due to prescription opioid analgesics.
- The REMS program requires that training be made available to all healthcare providers (HCPs) who are involved in the management of patients with pain, including nurses and pharmacists (FDA, n.d.).

Substance Abuse and Mental Health Services Administration (SAMHSA)

- SAMHSA's Center for Substance Abuse Prevention (CSAP) provides national leadership in the development of policies, programs, and services to prevent the onset of substance misuse. SAMHSA's Center for Substance Abuse Treatment (CSAT) promotes community-based substance abuse treatment and recovery services for in every community. CSAT provides leadership to improve access, reduce barriers, and promote high quality, effective treatment and recovery services.

- SAMHSA's Evidence-Based Practices Resource (EBPR) Center works to provide communities, clinicians, policymakers, and others in the field with the information they need to incorporate evidence-based practices in their communities for prevention, treatment, and recovery services (SAMHSA, 2020).

Agency for Healthcare Research and Quality (AHRQ)

- The AHRQ, along with other HHS Operating and Staff Divisions, supports the HHS 5-Point Strategy to Combat the Opioids Crisis, which includes: better OUD prevention, treatment, and recovery services, better data, better research, better targeting of overdose-reversing drugs, and better pain management. Of these, AHRQ focus areas are: better substance use disorder prevention, treatment, and recovery services; better data; and better research.
- AHRQ is supporting primary care practices in delivering evidence-based MOUD for opioid abuse in rural areas.
- In 2016, the AHRQ invested about $12 million over 3 years in a series of grants that are exploring and testing solutions aimed at overcoming barriers to the use of MOUD in rural primary care settings.
- The grants are also providing MOUD access using innovative technology to more than 20,000 individuals. Such strategies include patient-controlled smart phone apps, and remote training and expert consultation using a telehealth program that began with AHRQ support, to link specialists at an academic hub to primary care providers working in rural communities (AHRQ, 2018).

Department of Defense (DoD)

- Veterans Administration/Department of Defense (VA/DoD) has Clinical Practice Guidelines for Opioid Therapy (OT). The guidelines describe the critical decision points in the management of opioid therapy for chronic pain and provides comprehensive evidence-based recommendations incorporating current information and practices for practitioners throughout the DoD and VA Health Care systems.
- The DoD's Defense Health Agency-Procedural Instruction (DHA-PI) is a dual effort between the Pain Management Clinical Support Service and the Clinical Communities to achieve the stated purpose through implementation of the Military Health System (MHS) Stepped Care Model.
- The DoD ensures the incorporation of Defense and Veterans Pain Rating Scale (DVPRS) and Pain Assessment Screening Tool and Outcomes Registry (PASTOR) as pain measurement and outcomes tools. It ensures that MHS GENESIS provides alerts and other clinical support tools to assist clinical personnel in evidence-based pain management and safe opioid prescribing.
- The agency provides virtual Opioid Prescriber Safety Training (OPST) and other designated trainings regarding opioid prescribing and patient education on opioid risks.
- The agency delivers laboratory support to assure urine drug testing for screening and confirmation of controlled substances for those on long-term opioid therapy or other patients at risk for opioid use disorder to maximize patient safety (VA, 2017).

Veterans Affairs (VA)

- The VA emphasizes the safe and responsible use of prescription opioids in the context of a broader transition from a biomedical to a biopsychosocial model of pain care.
- The VA announced it has successfully reduced prescription opioid use in patients within the VA healthcare system by 64%, from more than 679,000 veterans in fiscal year 2012 to 247,000 in fiscal year 2020 through the 3rd quarter.
- The VA achieved this reduction by emphasizing the safe and responsible use of prescription opioids and transforming the treatment of chronic pain using alternative therapies in place of or in conjunction with pain medication.
- Through its Opioid Overdose Education & Naloxone Distribution program, the VA has distributed more than 416,000 prescriptions of naloxone, a life-saving medication used to block the effects of a potentially fatal opioid overdose.
- Under the Drug "Take Back" program, veterans have safely returned approximately 192.3 tons of medications.
- Specially trained VA pharmacists have conducted more than 55,000 outreach visits with VA staff on opioid safety, opioid overdose and naloxone distribution, and MOUD.
- The VA Opioid Overdose Education & Naloxone Distribution (OEND) program aims to reduce harm and risk of life-threatening, opioid-related overdose and deaths among veterans. Key components of the OEND program include education and training regarding opioid overdose prevention, recognition of opioid overdose, opioid overdose rescue response, and the issue of naloxone kits. The VA Academic Detailing Service has worked with Office of Mental Health Operations to produce patient education brochures for overdose prevention, overdose recognition, and instructional guides for the naloxone products (VA, 2020).

Department of Agriculture (USDA)

- The USDA is committed to being a strong partner to rural communities on a number of fronts: through program resources for prevention, treatment, and recovery opportunities for those in need; through program resources to help rural communities address many of the deeper, systemic, and long-term issues that make these places vulnerable to the opioid crisis, through the creation of essential tools for rural leaders to use to understand the impact and cause(s) of the crisis in their community; and tools to understand what federal resources are available to help support grassroots strategies to address this crisis.
- The Rural Resource Guide to Help Address Substance Use Disorder and Opioid Misuse is the second tool announced in the USDA's Community Opioid Misuse Toolbox—a suite of essential tools supporting grassroots strategies to address the opioid epidemic. Earlier, the USDA launched the Community Assessment Tool, an interactive database to help community leaders assess how and why the opioid epidemic is impacting their regions. The USDA's Community Opioid Misuse Toolbox is free and available to the public (USDA, n.d.).

Agency for International Development (USAID)

- Methadone Maintenance Therapy (MMT) refers to the use of methadone to treat OUD. Since 2015, USAID's Sustainable HIV Response from Technical Assistance (SHIFT) activity has made significant strides in convincing local authorities to scale up MMT as a cost-effective, evidence-based, humane means to prevent HIV transmission and treat drug abuse.
- SHIFT has provided coaching and advocacy, with a consistent emphasis on sustainability in Nghe An and Dien Bien provinces in Vietnam. This work has resulted in achieving a sustainability milestone: Both provinces recently committed to enroll a total of 7,400 MMT patients by 2019, a 90% increase from the 3,927 patients currently enrolled.
- In Kenya, USAID formulated a strategy to make evidence-based Opioid Substitution Therapy (OST), MOUD, Needle and Syringe Program (NSP), and referral and linking to HIV Testing and Counselling (HTC) and Antiretroviral Therapy (ART) services available, accessible, and scalable to reach large numbers of people with infectious diseases (U.S. Agency for International Development, 2017).

Drug Enforcement Administration (DEA)

- The Department of Justice and the DEA have proposed a "Safe Prescribing Plan" that seeks to "cut nationwide opioid prescription fills by one-third within three years," the proposal decreases manufacturing quotas for the six most frequently misused opioids for 2019 by an average 10% compared with the 2018 amount.
- The Proposed Aggregate Production Quotas for schedule I and II controlled substances published in the Federal Register reflects the total amount of controlled substances necessary to meet the country's medical, scientific, research, industrial, and export needs for the year and for the establishment and maintenance of reserve stocks.
- The DEA proposes to reduce the amount of fentanyl produced by 31%, hydrocodone by 19%, hydromorphone by 25%, oxycodone by 9%, and oxymorphone by 55%. Combined with morphine, the proposed quota would be a 53% decrease in the amount of allowable production of these opioids since 2016.
- The DEA's 360 Strategy responds to the heroin and prescription opioid pill crisis. The 360 Strategy takes an innovative, three-pronged approach to combating opioid use through: Coordinated Law Enforcement actions against drug cartels and heroin traffickers in specific communities; Diversion Control Enforcement actions against DEA registrants operating outside the law and long-term engagement with pharmaceutical drug manufacturers, wholesalers, pharmacies, and practitioners; and Community Outreach through local partnerships that empower communities.
- The DEA's narcotic treatment program registrants authorized to dispense narcotic drugs approved to treat opioid dependence would be authorized to implement a "mobile component" to their registration, eliminating the need for a separate DEA registration. This streamlined registration process will make it easier for providers to offer needed services in remote or underserved areas.

- A Federal bill required the DEA to provide drug manufacturers and distributors with access to anonymized information through the Automated Reports and Consolidated Orders System (ARCOS) will further help drug manufacturers and distributors to identify, report and stop suspicious orders of opioids and reduce diversion rates (DEA, 2018).

The Role of State Governments

States play an important role in the funding, oversite, and access to MOUD treatment services. Although the United States Congress passes laws and allocates funding, various federal agencies like SAMHSA administer grants and programs, and the DEA issues rules consistent with Congressional intent, States often serve as the conduit for federal grants and programs. For example, every state is given a baseline of federal substance use prevention and treatment dollars known as the federal Substance Abuse and Prevention Treatment Block Grant (SAPT). SAPT dollars are considered critical safety net funding for public prevention and treatment services (NASADAD, 2019). A minimum of 20% of every state's SAPT funding must be dedicated to prevention. In addition to administrating SAPT funding, the states play a critical role in supporting treatment services through their licensing procedures for SUD treatment facilities and reimbursement allocations, usually by setting state Medicaid/Medicare reimbursement rates. The states also play a central role in supporting the uptake of evidence-based OUD treatment services (SAMHSA, 2020). The states often contract with city and county health departments or programs (often not for profit but not always) to deliver prevention and treatment services in local communities. The states may also rely on programs or coalitions to help advance or defend opioid related laws and policies.

Non Governmental Policy Research and Advocacy Organizations

In addition to the various federal agencies working to address the opioid epidemic, there are policy research and policy advocacy nonprofit organizations. A few of these and their goals are described in the following pages based on the most current information from their websites and printed materials.

The Association of State and Territorial Health Officials (ASTHO) developed a framework recognizing the critical role of public health leaders and partners in carrying out a comprehensive, cross-sector response to the opioid epidemic (ASHTO, 2017). With cross-sector partnerships, states and territories can leverage four key strategies, including (1) training and education; (2) monitoring and surveillance; (3) treatment, recovery, and harm reduction; and (4) primary and overdose prevention. The association asserts that leadership from governmental and nongovernmental agencies across multiple levels (federal, state, and local) and sectors (health, public safety, corrections, drug control, and education) is needed to comprehensively address the epidemic within states and territories. They also advocate for resources that are critical to the full implementation of this framework.

The National Association of City and County Health (NACCHO) recognizes prescription and illicit opioid misuse as a significant public health threat and national emergency, as well as the critical role that local health departments play in responding to the nation's opioid epidemic. The NACCHO supports local health departments to respond to the opioid epidemic through the implementation of evidence-based policies and programs for the prevention and treatment of OUD. Local strategies encompass improvements in surveillance and monitoring, increases in prevention and education, promotion of appropriate opioid prescribing practices, and improvement and expansion of treatment and recovery services for OUD. As the opioid epidemic progresses, the NACCHO continues to provide new resources and tools to support local health departments as they build a response within their own communities (NACCHO, 2020).

The National Academy for State Health Policy (NASHP) is working with states to develop a "no-wrong-door" approach to OUD treatment that prioritizes cross-systems policy. NASHP is providing tools and resources, which will be frequently expanded, with support from the Foundation for Opioid Response Efforts. Furthermore, NASHP emphasizes the ripple effect of the epidemic as it reaches beyond health systems to impact public safety and corrections, child protective services, and other state agencies and functions. However, the organization has identified state-level strategies that continue to show great promise. These include:

- Tracking opioid prescribing
- Expanding access to naloxone
- Increasing MOUD
- Engaging corrections
- Ensuring treatment in rural areas
- Expanding Medicaid (Purington, 2019)

The National Association of State Alcohol and Drug Abuse Directors (NASADAD) has as its basic purpose to foster and support the development of effective alcohol and other drug abuse prevention and treatment programs throughout every State. The NASADAD's objectives include: to aid putting research and awareness into practice, and to determine issues that warrant further research; to encourage both communication and collaboration with other associations dealing with substance abuse issues; to promote substance abuse prevention and treatment training; to endorse the formation of a model for quality assurance, outcomes, and performance; to construct public policy positions that will improve prevention and treatment services, along with increasing funding for those services.

Based in part on the findings of Ruhm's study of opioid deaths reported in the *American Journal of Preventive Medicine* (2017), the non-profit policy research group Altarum has recommended that policymakers focus on three areas:

- **Prevention.** Educating clinicians on the appropriate use of opioids and alternatives to treat pain; monitoring opioid prescribing and targeting high prescribers; encouraging benefits managers to explore drug tiers to create higher financial barriers to accessing opioids; and working with insurers to encourage alternatives for managing chronic pain.
- **Treatment.** Payment and delivery system reform to engage clinicians and community support services to better manage the needs of people with OUDs; encouraging employers to provide value-based insurance design features to remove barriers to treatment.

- **Recovery.** In-depth understanding of the length of time to help people with OUDs to recover from the dependency and to facilitate access to the essential local support services that are key to more successful recovery rates (Altarum, 2018).

National Policy Recommendations

In 2018, The National Academy of Medicine and the Aspen Institute launched the Action Collaborative on Countering the U.S. Opioid Epidemic. Focused on working across public, private, and nonprofit sectors, the Collaborative identified research gaps and the need for accelerated implementation of evidence-based responses to improve outcomes. Focus areas addressed through training, research, and publications include improving access to evidence-based OUD treatment, addressing the needs of priority populations, and best practices in the management of chronic noncancer pain. Priority recommendations include:

1. Pain Management
   - Training and education for clinicians to support a patient-centered, coordinated interprofessional approach to acute and chronic pain management and SUD.
2. Evidence-Based Treatment
   - Promote guidelines and standards for opioid prescribing for acute and chronic pain that align clinical implementation, promote best practices, and support limited and appropriate prescribing.
   - Improve access to quality treatment through dissemination of identified best practices for OUD prevention, treatment, and recovery services including guidance on implementation, scaling, and sustaining high-quality services and outcomes.
   - Identify critical research gaps and address data access needs to support appropriate data sharing, quality metrics, and research (National Academy of Medicine, 2021).

After the launch of its Action Collaborative, the National Academies of Science, Engineering, and Medicine in 2019 published *Medications for Opioid Use Disorder Save Lives*, which identified barriers to increased uptake of MOUD. Barriers included: stigma, lack of provider education, and the restrictive MOUD regulatory environment (NAM, 2019). In July of 2020, the Action Collaborative's treatment-focused working group published a discussion paper aimed at identifying strategies to address these barriers and improve access to care. This report breaks down provider, institutional, regulatory, financial, and other barriers identifying specific actions that congress, federal agencies, the states, public and private payors, and treatment systems can take to respond to the national opioid crisis (Madras et al., 2020). Key strategies include:

Equitable treatment access:

- Develop and implement a national antistigma campaign.
- Address complex patient needs and expedite access to MOUD, by funding innovative models that address social determinants of health and racial and geographic disparities in access to services.

- Consult people with OUD to improve services and fund research on patient engagement and motivation for treatment.
- Enforce mental health parity laws.
- Expand Medicaid, provide medication coverage in detention, and facilitate health coverage for incarcerated populations.
- Improve insurance coverage and access to all three MOUD medications.

Provider training and workforce development:

- Require clinician training in screening, diagnosis, and treatment of OUD.
- Train more addiction specialists and encourage practice in underserved communities.

Regulatory and systems barriers to access, data sharing, and research:

- Reform legal, training, and nurse practitioner restrictions to expand access to MOUD.
- Eliminate preemptive state laws that add additional barriers to MOUD access and reduce utilization policies by public and private payors that restrict access to MOUD treatment.
- Create quality measures for OUD treatment and promote evidence-based practice through funding and technical assistance.
- Revise restrictions and fund research on data-sharing programs and tools to improve access to overdose mortality and other opioid-related health outcomes (Madras et al., 2020).

Discussion Questions

1. Identify and describe key federal agencies involved in opioids policy and regulation.
2. Discuss why policy is an important part of the overall strategy to mitigate the opioids epidemic.
3. Describe and discuss the role of health systems in the above-mentioned strategy.

References

Abraham, A. J., Andrews, C. M., Grogan, C. M., D'Aunno, T., Humphreys, K. N., Pollack, H. A., & Friedmann, P. D. (2017). The Affordable Care Act Transformation of Substance Use Disorder Treatment. *American Journal of Public Health, 107*(1), 31–32.

Agency for Healthcare Research and Quality. (2018). Building bridges between research and practice: Opiods. Retrieved from https://www.ahrq.gov/sites/default/files/wysiwyg/topics/impact-opioid-final.pdf

Altarum. (2018). Economic toll of opioid crisis in U.S. exceeded $1 trillion since 2001. Retrieved from https://altarum.org/news/economic-toll-opioid-crisis-us-exceeded-1-trillion-2001

American Hospital Association. (2019). 2019 AHA hospital statistics. Retrieved from https://www.aha.org/statistics/fast-facts-us-hospitals

American Society of Addiction Medicine. (2015). The ASAM national practice guideline for the use of medications in the treatment of addiction involving opioid use. Retrieved from https://www.asam.org/docs/default-source/practice-support/guidelines-and-consensus-docs/asam-national-practice-guideline-supplement.pdf

Association of State and Territorial Health Officials. (2017). State opioid response plans for 2018. Retrieved from http://www.astho.org/StatePublicHealth/State-Opioid-Response-Plans-for-2018/12-21-17/

Blevins, C. E., Rawat, N., & Stein, M. D. (2018). Gaps in the substance use disorder treatment referral process: Provider perceptions. *Journal of Addiction Medicine, 12*(4), 273–277.

Bonnie, R. J., Ford, M. A., & Phillips, J. K. (Eds.). (2017). *Pain management and the opioid epidemic: Balancing societal and individual benefits and risks of prescription opioid use.* Washington, DC: The National Academies Press. doi:10.17226 /24781

Campbell, J., & Rooney, S. (2018). *A time-release history of the opioid epidemic.* Cham, Switzerland: Springer.

Centers for Disease Control and Prevention. (n.d.). Understanding the epidemic. Retrieved from https://www.cdc.gov/drugoverdose/epidemic/index.html

Centers for Disease Control and Prevention. (2017). Opioid prescribing. *CDC Vital Signs.* Retrieved from https://www.cdc.gov/vitalsigns/pdf/2017-07-vitalsigns.pdf

The Center for Health Affairs. (2018). The Northeast Ohio Hospital opioid consortium. Retrieved from https://www.neohospitals.org/Community-Outreach/~/~/link.aspx?_id=22 FF8E35F4724C1E95DCFC745201AE7A&_z=z

Center for Substance Abuse Treatment. (1997). A guide to substance abuse services for primary care clinicians. Rockville (MD): Substance Abuse and Mental Health Services Administration (US). (Treatment Improvement Protocol (TIP) Series, No. 24.) Chapter 5—Specialized Substance Abuse Treatment Programs. Available from: https://www.ncbi.nlm.nih.gov/books/NBK64815/

Center for Substance Abuse Treatment. (2005). Substance abuse treatment for persons with co-occurring disorders. Rockville (MD): Substance Abuse and Mental Health Services Administration (US). (Treatment Improvement Protocol (TIP) Series, No. 42.) Available from: https://www.ncbi.nlm.nih.gov/books/NBK64184/figure/A74172/

Chen, Q., Larochelle, M. R., Weaver, D. T., Lietz, A. P., Mueller, P. P., Mercaldo, S., . . . Chhatwal, J. (2019). Prevention of prescription opioid misuse and projected overdose deaths in the United States. *JAMA Network Open, 2*(2), e187621. doi:10.1001/jamanetworkopen.2018.7621

The Council of Economic Advisers. (2017). The underestimated cost of the opioid crisis. Retrieved from https://www.whitehouse.gov/sites/whitehouse.gov/files/images/The%20Underestimated %20Cost%20of%20the%20Opioid%20Crisis.pdf

Commonwealth Fund Opioids 2020 https://www.commonwealthfund.org/trending/opioid-crisis

D'Onofrio, G., McCormack, R. P., & Hawk, K. (2018). Emergency departments—a 24/7/365 option for combating the opioid crisis. *New England Journal of Medicine, 379*(26), 2487–2490. doi:10.1056/NEJMp1811988

Dowell, D., Haegerich, T. M., & Chou, R. (2016). CDC guideline for prescribing opioids for chronic pain—United States, 2016. *JAMA, 315*(15), 1624–1645.

The General Hospital Corporation. (2018). MGPO task force. Retrieved from https://www.massgeneral.org/opioid-task-force.aspx

Goldner, E. M., Lusted, A., Roerecke, M., Rehm, J., & Fischer, B. (2014). Prevalence of Axis-1 psychiatric (with focus on depression and anxiety) disorder and symptomatology among non-medical prescription opioid users in substance use treatment: Systematic review and meta-analyses. *Addictive Behaviors, 39*(3), 520–531.

Hasegawa, K., Espinola, J. A., Brown, D. F., & Camargo, C. A. (2014). Trends in US emergency department visits for opioid overdose, 1993–2010. *Pain Medicine, 15*(10), 1765–1770.

Health Resources & Services Administration. (n.d.-a). FY 2019 Integrated behavioral health services (IBHS) supplemental funding (HRSA-19-100). Retrieved from https://bphc.hrsa.gov /qualityimprovement/clinicalquality/substance-use-disorder-primary-care-integration

Health Resources & Services Administration. (n.d.-b). Substance use disorders and primary care integration. Retrieved from https://bphc.hrsa.gov/qualityimprovement/clinicalquality /substance-use-disorder-primary-care-integration

Indian Health Services. (n.d.). Opioid use disorder and pain. Retrieved from https://www.ihs.gov /opioids

The Johns Hopkins Health System. (2018). About Johns Hopkins. Retrieved from https://www .hopkinsmedicine.org/about/index.html

Johnson, J. A. (2018). *Medical Social Science and Systems Thinking Perspectives on the U.S. Opioid Epidemic.* New Orleans, LA: National Social Science Association Conference.

Johnson, J. A., & Anderson, D. E. (2017). *Systems thinking for health organizations, leadership, and policy* (pp. 101–108). Austin, TX: Sentia Publishing.

Johnson, J. A., Anderson, D. E., & Rossow, C. C. (2019). *Health systems thinking.* Burlington, MA: Jones & Bartlett Learning.

Johnson, J. A., & Davey, K. S. (2021). *Essentials of managing public health organizations.* Burlington, MA: Jones & Bartlett Learning.

Johnson, J. A., & Rossow, C. C. (2019). *Health organizations* (2nd ed.). Burlington, MA: Jones & Bartlett Learning.

Johnson, J. A., Stoskopf, C. H., & Shi, L. (2018). *Comparative health systems: A global perspective.* Burlington, MA: Jones & Bartlett Learning.

Kaiser Family Foundation. (2020). Status of state action on the Medicaid expansion decision. Retrieved from https://www.kff.org/health-reform/state-indicator/state-activity-around-expanding-medicaid-under-the-affordable-care-act

Kelly, T. M., Daley, D. C. (2013). Integrated treatment of substance use and psychiatric disorders. *Social Work in Public Health,* 28(3–4):388–406. doi:10.1080/19371918.2013.774673.

Krawczyk, N., Picher, C. E., Feder, K. A., & Saloner, B. (2017). Only one in twenty justice-referred adults in specialty treatment for opioid use receive methadone or buprenorphine. *Health Affairs, 36*(12), 2046–2053.

Leshner, A. I., & Mancher, M. (Eds.). (2019). *Medications for opioid use disorder save lives.* Washington, DC: The National Academies Press. doi:10.17226/25310

Madras, B. K., Ahmad, N. J., Wen, J., Sharfstein, J., & the Prevention, Treatment, and Recovery Working Group of the Action Collaborative on Countering the U.S. Opioid Epidemic. (2020). Improving access to evidence-based medical treatment for opioid use disorder: Strategies to address key barriers within treatment systems. *National Academy of Medicine Perspectives.* Retrieved from https://doi.org/10.31478/202004b

NACCHO (2020) Opioid Epidemic Tool Kit. National Association of City and County Health Officers. https://www.naccho.org/programs/community-health/injury-and-violence/opioid-epidemic/local-health-departments-and-the-opioid-epidemic-a-toolkit

National Academy of Medicine, Action Collaborative on Clinician Well-Being and Resilience. (2021). Guiding principles. Retrieved from https://nam.edu/programs/action-collaborative-on-countering-the-u-s-opioid-epidemic/opioid-ac-goals-and-guiding-principles/

National Academies of Sciences, Engineering, and Medicine. (2019). More than 100 organization join the National Academy of Medicine in countering the opioid epidemic [News release]. Retrieved from https://www.nationalacademies.org/news/2019/04/more-than-100-organizations-join-the-national-academy-of-medicine-in-countering-the-opioid-epidemic

National Academies of Sciences, Engineering, and Medicine. (2018). *Integrating responses at the intersection of opioid use disorder and infectious disease epidemics.* Washington, DC: National Academies Press. doi:10.17226/25153

National Association of State Alcohol and Drug Abuse Directors (2019). Substance Abuse Prevention and Treatment Block (SAPT) Grant. Retrieved from file:///C:/Users/lfrazier/OneDrive%20-%20Advocates%20for%20Human%20Potential/LF/Opioids%20and%20Pop%20Health/SAPT-Block-Grant-Fact-Sheet-March-2019.pdf

National HIV Curriculum. (2021). CAGE-AID Questionnaire. Retrieved from https://www.hiv.uw.edu/page/substance-use/cage-aid

National Institute on Drug Abuse. (2020). Opioid overdose crisis. Retrieved from: https://www.drugabuse.gov/drugs-abuse/opioids/opioid-overdose-crisis

National Institute on Drug Abuse. (2021). NIDA-Modified ASSIST (NM ASSIST). Retrieved from https://archives.drugabuse.gov/nmassist/

National Institutes of Health. (2021). NIH HEAL Initiative research plan. Retrieved from https://www.nih.gov/research-training/medical-research-initiatives/heal-initiative/heal-initiative-research-plan

Operation UNITE. (2018). About operation UNITE. Retrieved from https://operationunite.org/about/

Overmountain Recovery. (2018). Substance-abuse treatment clinic in Johnson City, TN. Retrieved from https://www.overmountainrecovery.org/

The Patient Protection and Affordable Care Act. (2010). Retrieved from Congress: https://www.govinfo.gov/content/pkg/PLAW-111publ148/pdf/PLAW-111publ148.pdf

The Pew Charitable Trusts. (2019). Substance use disorder treatment policy recommendations for the state of Delaware. Retrieved from https://ltgov.delaware.gov/wp-content/uploads/sites/27/2019/04/Delaware-Recommendations-for-OUD-Treatment-Expansion-Embargoed-Final-Draft.pdf

Purington, K. (2019). Tackling the opioid crisis: What state strategies are working? Retrieved from https://www.nashp.org/tackling-the-opioid-crisis-what-state-strategies-are-working

Ruhm C. J. (2017). Geographic variation in opioid and heroin involved drug poisoning mortality rates. *American Journal of Preventive Medicine, 53*(6), 745–753

Ries, R. K., Fiellin, D. A., Miller, S. C., & Saitz, R. (2019). *The ASAM principles of addiction medicine* (6th ed.). Netherlands: Wolters Kluwer.

Robeznieks, A. (2018). Remove barriers to opioid-use disorder treatment. Retrieved from https://www.ama-assn.org/delivering-care/opioids/ama-remove-barriers-opioid-use-disorder-treatment

Rollman, J., Heyward, J., Olson, L., Lurie, P., Sharfstein, J., & Alexander, C. (2019). Assessment of the FDA risk evaluation and mitigation strategy for transmucosal immediate-release fentanyl products. *JAMA, 321*(7), 676–685.

Saitz, R. (2014). Screening and brief intervention for unhealthy drug use: Little or no efficacy. *Frontiers in Psychiatry, 5*, 1–5.

Saloner, B., & Maclean, J. C. (2020). Specialty Substance Use Disorder Treatment Admissions Steadily Increased In The Four Years After Medicaid Expansion. *Health Affairs, 39*(3), 453–461.

Schieber, L. Z., Guy., G. P., Seth, P., Young, R., Mattson, C., Mikosz, C., & Schieber, R. A. (2019). Trends and patterns of geographic variation in opioid prescribing practices by state, United States, 2006–2017. *JAMA Network Open, 2*(3):e190665. doi:10.1001/jamanetworkopen.2019.0665

Substance Abuse and Mental Health Services Administration. (2015). Federal guidelines for opioid treatment programs. HHS Publication No. (SMA) PEP15-FEDGUIDEOTP. Rockville, MD: Substance Abuse and Mental Health Services Administration. https://store.samhsa.gov/sites/default/files/d7/priv/pep15-fedguideotp.pdf

Substance Abuse and Mental Health Services Administration. (2016). Results from the 2016 national survey on drug use and health: Detailed tables. Rockville, MD.

Substance Abuse and Mental Health Services Administration. (2017). Substance abuse prevention and treatment block grant. Retrieved from SAMHSA: https://www.samhsa.gov/grants/block-grants/sabg

Substance Abuse and Mental Health Services Administration. (2020). Prevention of substance use and mental disorders. Retrieved from https://www.samhsa.gov/find-help/prevention

Substance Abuse and Mental Health Services Administration, U.S. Department of Health and Human Services. (2018). National survey of substance abuse treatment services (N-SSATS): 2017. Rockville, MD.

Substance use disorder prevention that promotes opioid recovery and treatment for patients and communities act. (2018). Retrieved from https://www.congress.gov/115/bills/hr6/BILLS-115hr6enr.pdf

The University of New Mexico. (2018). Project Echo: A revolution in medical education and care delivery. Retrieved from https://echo.unm.edu/

U.S. Agency for International Development. (2017). Nghe An and Dien Bien provinces achieve methadone treatment services sustainability milestone. Retrieved from https://www.usaid.gov/vietnam/program-updates/oct-2017-nghe-and-dien-bien-provinces-achieve-methadone-treatment-services

U.S. Department of Agriculture. (n.d.). Opioid misuse in rural America. Retrieved from https://www.usda.gov/topics/opioids

U.S. Department of Health and Human Services. (2018). Strategy to combat opioid abuse, misuse, and overdose: A framework based on the five point strategy.

U.S. Department of Health and Human Services, Office of the Surgeon General. (2018). Facing addiction in America: The Surgeon General's spotlight on opioids. Washington, DC: U.S.

Department of Health and Human Services. Retrieved from https://addiction.surgeongeneral.gov/sites/default/files/surgeon-generals-report.pdf

U.S. Department of Veterans Affairs. (2017). Management of opioid therapy (OT) for chronic pain. Retrieved from https://www.healthquality.va.gov/guidelines/pain/cot/index.asp

U.S. Department of Veterans Affairs. (2020). VA reduces prescription opioid use by 64% during past eight years. Retrieved from https://www.va.gov/opa/pressrel/pressrelease.cfm?id=5492

U.S. Drug Enforcement Administration. (2018). Justice Department, DEA propose significant opioid manufacturing reduction in 2019 [Press release]. Retrieved from https://www.dea.gov/press-releases/2018/08/16/justice-department-dea-propose-significant-opioid-manufacturing-reduction

U.S. Food and Drug Administration. (n.d.). Opioid analgesic risk evaluation and mitigation strategy (REMS). Retrieved from https://www.fda.gov/drugs/information-drug-class/opioid-analgesic-risk-evaluation-and-mitigation-strategy-rems

VanHouten, J., Rudd, R., Ballesteros, M., & Mack, K. (2019). Drug overdose deaths among women aged 30–64 years—United States, 1999–2017. *Morbidity and Mortality Weekly Report, 68*(1), 1–5. Retrieved from https://www.cdc.gov/mmwr/volumes/68/wr/pdfs/mm6801a1-H.pdf

Volkow, N. D., & McLellan, A. T. (2016). Opioid abuse in chronic pain — misconceptions and mitigation strategies. *The New England Journal of Medicine*, (374), 1253–1263. doi:10.1056/NEJMra1507771

Volkow, N. D., Jones, E. B., Einstein, E. B., (2019). Prevention and treatment of opioid misuse and addiction. *JAMA, 76*(2), 208–216. doi:10.1001/jamapsychiatry.2018.3126

Vowles, K. E., McEntee, M. L., Julnes, P. S., Frohe, T., Ney, J. P., & Van Der Goes, D. N. (2015). Rates of opioid misuse, abuse, and addiction in chronic pain: A systematic review and data synthesis. *Pain, 156*(4), 569–576. doi:10.1097/01.j.pain.0000460357.01998.f1

World Health Organization. (2011). Health systems strengthening glossary. Retrieved from https://www.who.int/healthsystems/Glossary_January2011.pdf

Zhu, W., Chernew, M. E., Sherry, T. B., & Maestas, M. (2019). Initial opioid prescriptions among U.S. commercially insured patients, 2012–2017. *The New England Journal of Medicine, 380*(11), 1043–1052. doi:10.1056/NEJMsa1807069

Glossary

A

Acute Pain Pain that starts suddenly and lasts less than three months. Acute pain has a known cause, usually from an injury or surgery that gets better as the body heals.

Affordable Care Act (ACA) The Patient Protection and Affordable Care Act (aka: the ACA or Obamacare) PUBLIC LAW 111–148—MAR. 23, 2010. The ACA makes affordable health insurance available to more people, eliminates preconditions as a reason to be denied insurance, expands Medicaid and more. The law also outlines benefits and responsibilities for employers and other organizations, including coverage parity for treatment of mental health and substance use disorders.

Analgesics Pain relieving medications including over-the-counter medications like acetaminophen (Tylenol®) or ibuprofen (Advil®) and prescription opioids.

B

Behavioral Therapies for substance use disorders Behavioral health counseling or psychotherapy treatments that are evidence based ways of helping people manage physical, mental health, and substance use disorders using talk therapy.

Benzodiazepines A type of sedative medication prescribed for anxiety. Benzodiazepines (or "benzos") raise the level of the inhibitory neurotransmitter GABA in the brain, which has a calming effect. Some common benzodiazepines include diazepam (Valium), alprazolam (Xanax), and clonazepam (Klonopin).

Buprenorphine A medication approved by the U.S. Food and Drug Administration (FDA) in 2002 to treat opioid use disorders (OUD). Buprenorphine is the first medication to treat OUD that can be prescribed or dispensed in primary healthcare services. Primary care prescribers (physicians, physician assistants, and nurse practitioners) must complete specialized training to receive a buprenorphine waiver certification to be eligible to prescribe. In addition, buprenorphine can also be administered at SAMHSA-certified opioid treatment programs (OTPs).

C

CDC Guidelines for Prescribing Opioids Published in 2016, these guidelines provide recommendations for primary care clinicians prescribing opioids for chronic pain that is not for the treatment of active cancer, palliative care, or end-of-life care. The CDC published a subsequent statement instructing providers that abrupt termination of opioid prescriptions for those with prolonged exposure was not in keeping with the guidelines or sound medical practice. https://www.cdc.gov/media/releases/2019/s0424-advises-misapplication-guideline-prescribing-opioids.html

Centers for Disease Control and Prevention (CDC) The national health assessment, promotion, prevention, protection, and preparedness agency. CDC leads science-based, data-driven responses to protect the public's health.

Centers for Medicare & Medicaid Services (CMS) CMS is part of the US Department of Health and Human Services (HHS). CMS was created in 1977 to administer the Medicare and Medicaid programs.

Chronic pain Pain that lasts three months or more and is caused by a disease or condition, inflammation, injury, medical procedures, or unknown factors.

Cirrhosis Cirrhosis is a chronic condition in which the liver is scarred and permanently damaged. Common causes of cirrhosis include alcoholic liver disease and chronic hepatitis C and B (HCV, HBV).

Clinical Trial A research study that assigns human subjects to one or more interventions (which may include placebo or other control) to evaluate the effects of the interventions on health-related behavioral or biomedical outcomes.

Cocaine An addictive stimulant drug made from the leaves of the coca plant.

Controlled Substances Act (CSA) The Comprehensive Drug Abuse Prevention and Control Act of 1970, Pub.L. 91–513, 84 Stat. 1236, enacted October 27, 1970. Known as the Controlled Substances Act, places all regulated substances under federal law into one of five schedules.

D

Diagnostic and Statistical Manual of Mental Disorders, 5th Edition (DSM-5) Published by the American Psychological Association, the manual outlines diagnostic criteria and treatment recommendations for health care providers treating mental health and substance use disorders.

Drug Diversion When prescription medicines are obtained for use beyond medical indication.

Drug Enforcement Agency (DEA) Federal law enforcement agency within the U.S. Department of Justice, responsible for enforcing the controlled substances laws and regulations of the United States.

Drug Misuse The use of prescription medications in a manner other than as directed by a doctor.

Drug Scheduling The U.S. Drug Enforcement Administration (DEA) is charged with enforcement of the Controlled Substances Act pertaining to the manufacture, distribution, and dispensing of legally produced controlled substances. Five different schedules are used to rank drugs according to medical use and risk to human health.

E

Epidemic An increase in the number of cases of a disease above what is normally expected for that population in that area.

Evidence-based Treatment Evidence-based treatment includes behavioral health, medication, and other treatment interventions that have been scientifically shown to have positive outcomes through high-quality research.

F

Federal Agencies Federal agencies are government organizations set up for a specific purpose such as preventing or mitigating the opioid epidemic.

Fentanyl A powerful synthetic opioid analgesic that is 50 to 100 times more potent than morphine. In medicine, it is used to treat surgical patients with severe pain or to manage acute pain. In its prescription form, fentanyl is known by such names as Actiq®, Duragesic®, and Sublimaze®.

Food and Drug Administration (FDA) A part of the U.S. Department of Health and Human Services, the agency protects the public health by assuring the safety, effectiveness, and security of drugs, vaccines, and other biological products and medical devices.

G

Good Samaritan Law These laws grant varying degrees of immunity from prosecution for drug-related offenses by encouraging both victims and witnesses of an overdose to call 911. Forty states and the District of Columbia have enacted Good Samaritan laws specific to opioid overdose.

H

Harm Reduction A public health strategy to reduce the most immediate and consequential harms even if the strategy does not eliminate all potential risks or harms. Harm reduction strategies for opioid use include syringe service programs, safe injection sites, access to naloxone, and easy access to treatment and healthcare services.

HCV Hepatitis C is a liver infection caused by the hepatitis C virus (HCV). Hepatitis C is spread through contact with blood from an infected person. Some HCV infections convert to a long-term chronic infection that can be fatal. In 2013, a new class of medications was developed that allows patients to be cured of infection after two months of continuous medication treatment.

Heroin An illicit opioid drug made from morphine, a natural substance taken from the seed pod of opium poppy plants.

HIV Stands for human immunodeficiency virus. HIV is a chronic, medically manageable infection that weakens a person's immune system by destroying important cells that fight disease and infection. No effective cure exists for HIV, but the infection can be managed with medication.

I

Iatrogenic Disease that is the result of diagnostic procedures or therapeutic treatments offered under medical care.

Illicit drugs The nonmedical use of a variety of "illegal" drugs.

Incidence The occurrence of new cases of disease or injury in a population over a specified period of time.

Indian Health Service (IHS) The agency within the U.S. Department of Health and Human Services responsible for providing federal health services to American Indians and Alaska Natives. IHS provides health resources for approximately 2.6 million American Indians and Alaska Natives of 574 federally recognized tribes in 37 states.

International Classification of Diseases, 10th Edition (ICD-10) Published by the World Health Organization, the International Statistical Classification of Diseases and Related Health Problems outlines diagnostic codes for medical professionals. It is used by the Centers for Medicare and Medicaid Services (CMS) for reporting and reimbursement.

M

Medicaid Medicaid is the shared federal/state program that helps with medical costs for some people with limited income and resources.

Medicare Medicare is the federally supported U.S. health insurance program for people aged 65 or older.

Medication for Opioid Use Disorders (MOUD) Medications approved by the Food and Drug Administration (FDA) to treat opioid use disorders.

Medication-Assisted Therapies/Treatment (MAT) Medications approved by the Food and Drug Administration (FDA) to treat opioid use disorders. Term is slowly being replaced by Medication for Opioid Use Disorders (MOUD).

Methadone A medication used to treat Opioid Use Disorders (OUD). Methadone is a long-acting full opioid agonist that reduces opioid craving and withdrawal and blocks the effects of opioids.

Methadone Maintenance Treatment (MMT) has been offered by federally certified Opioid Treatment Programs (OTPs) since the 1950s. Individuals with a recent OUD diagnosis receive a daily dose of methadone (liquid or wafer) along with behavioral treatment. Take-home doses of medication are available as patients progress through the phases of treatment.

Morphine A non-synthetic opioid made from opium. Very effective for pain relief but holds high potential for abuse. Prescribed formulations include Kadian®, MS-Contin®, Oramorph SR®, MSIR®, RMS®, and Roxanol®.

Morphine Milligram Equivalents (MME) The equivalent measure of milligrams of morphine contained in a dose of any prescribed opioid.

Mortality Rate A measure of the frequency of death in a defined population over a specified period of time.

Mu-opioid Receptor (μOR) Mu opioid receptors mediate opioid pleasure effects and provide a reinforcing role for continued opioid use or indirect activation.

N

Naloxone A powerful opioid antagonist medication designed to rapidly reverse opioid overdose by binding and blocking opioid receptors. Naloxone should be prescribed to patients with a history of overdose or high dose opioid prescriptions (≥50 MME per day).

Naltrexone A medication to treat both opioid use (OUD) and alcohol use disorders (AUD). Naltrexone can be prescribed and administered by any practitioner licensed to prescribe medications. It is available in pill form for AUD or as Extended Release Injectable Naltrexone (ERIN) for either an AUD or OUD. Development of a Risk Evaluation and Mitigation Strategy (REMS) is required for the long-acting injectable formulation to ensure that the benefits of the drug outweigh the risks.

Narcotic From the Greek word for "stupor," "narcotic" refers to opium, opium derivatives, as well as their semi-synthetic substitutes.

National Association of County and City Health Officials (NACCHO) NACCHO is a member association that represents 3,000 local health departments across the United States. Founded in 1965, it was formerly titled the National Association of County Health Officials.

National Association of State Substance Abuse and Drug Abuse Directors (NASADAD) A private, not-for-profit educational, scientific, and informational organization. Incorporated in 1971 to serve State Drug Agency Directors. Membership was expanded to include State Alcoholism Agency Directors in 1978.

National Institute on Drug Abuse (NIDA) The lead federal agency supporting scientific research on drug use and its consequences. NIDA is one of 27 Institutes and Centers of the National Institutes of Health (NIH).

National Survey on Drug Use and Health (NSDUH) Formerly titled National Household Survey on Drug Abuse, NSDUH is a major source of statistical information on the use of illicit drugs, alcohol, tobacco, and mental health issues in the U.S. population of people aged 12 and older.

O

Opiates Refers to natural opioids such as heroin, morphine, and codeine.

Opioid Agonist Opioid agonists are medications that bind to the same receptors that other opioids activate. By binding to the receptors in the brain (and central nervous system), agonist medications eliminate withdrawal symptoms and relieve craving. Agonists occupy and activate opioid receptors more slowly than other opioids. Agonists (such as methadone) do not produce euphoria among opioid-dependent persons.

Opioid Antagonist Opioid antagonists work by blocking activation of opioid receptors. Agonist medications block other opioids from the opioid receptor and can cause withdrawal. They do not produce euphoria and do not decrease cravings. Naltrexone is an example of an opioid antagonist.

Opioid Dependence Occurs when the body adjusts its normal functioning to accommodate regular opioid use. Unpleasant physical symptoms may occur when opioids are stopped.

Opioid Policy Opioid policy is the collective policy, regulatory, and statutory rules, regulations, laws, and guidelines promulgated by federal, state, and local government agencies to address the opioid epidemic.

Opioid Overdose An opioid overdose occurs when an individual takes a higher dose of opioid than they can tolerate. Opioid overdose can be life-threatening and requires immediate emergency attention. When used beyond medical indication, persons using prescription opioid pain relievers or other prescription medications like methadone and buprenorphine can overdose.

Opioids A class of drugs that include illegal opioids like heroin, synthetic opioids such as fentanyl, and prescription pain relievers (used with and without a valid prescription) such as oxycodone (OxyContin®), hydrocodone (Vicodin®), codeine, and others.

Opioid Tolerance Occurs when a person using opioids begins to experience a reduced response to medication, requiring more opioids or a higher dose of opioids to experience the same effect.

Opioid Use Disorder (OUD) A pattern of opioid use that causes significant impairment or distress. Diagnosis is based on specific criteria such as unsuccessful attempts to cut down or control use, or use resulting in social problems, failure to fulfill obligations, among other criteria. OUD is preferred over other terms like "opioid abuse or dependence" or "opioid addiction." Diagnostic systems for medical and behavioral health personnel to make a diagnosis include the DSM-5 and the ICD-10.

Opium A highly addictive non-synthetic narcotic extracted from the poppy plant.

Overdose Injury to the body (poisoning) that happens when a drug is taken in excessive amounts. An overdose can be nonfatal or fatal.

Over the Counter (OTC) Medication Medicine that can be sold directly to people without a prescription (eg., Aspirin).

P

Partial Opioid Agonist Partial opioid agonists bind to the opioid receptors and activate them less strongly than full agonists. Partial agonists reduce cravings and withdrawal symptoms in persons with OUD without producing euphoria. Buprenorphine is an example of a partial opioid agonist.

Percutaneous (parenteral) Injection through the skin by needle (subcutaneous, intramuscular, or intravenous), by patch (transdermal), or by implantation.

Policy Context Policy context is the complex environment that influences how policy decisions are made as the result of simultaneous interactions between various stakeholders.

Policy Research Policy research is the process of conducting research on, or analysis of a fundamental social problem, such as the opioid epidemic, in order to provide policymakers with pragmatic, action-oriented recommendations for alleviating the problem.

Politics and Policy A policy is a statement of intent and is implemented as a procedure or protocol. Policies are generally adopted as regulations, laws, or practices.

Population Health A health outcome of a community or group of individuals, including the distribution of particular outcomes within the group.

Prescription Drug Monitoring Programs (PDMP) PDMPs are state-based database programs that collect information on controlled prescription drugs dispensed by pharmacies and (usually) prescribing providers. Some states require (mandate) that prescribers or their designees use the system.

Prescription Misuse Misuse of prescription drugs means taking a medication in a manner or at a dose or frequency other than prescribed, taking someone else's prescription, or taking a medication to feel euphoria (i.e., to get high). The term *nonmedical use* of prescription drugs also refers to misuse.

Prevalence Refers to the proportion of a population that has a particular disease or attribute at a specified point in time or over a specific period of time. Prevalence differs from incidence because it includes all cases, both new and preexisting, in the population at the specified time.

Public Health What we collectively do as a society to assure conditions in which individuals and communities can be healthy.

R

Racism The systemic oppression of a racial group to the social, economic, and political advantage of another.

Risk Evaluation and Mitigation Strategy (REMS) A drug safety program the U.S. Food and Drug Administration (FDA) requires for certain medications with serious safety concerns. REMS helps ensure that the benefits of using a medication outweigh risks.

Role of Health Systems A health system has the main aim to produce health in the population that is equitably distributed. Health systems are expected to treat people with dignity.

S

State Level Policy A state level policy occurs independent of or in collaboration with the federal government. Many opioid mitigation efforts involve every level of government.

Substance Abuse and Mental Health Service Administration (SAMHSA) Established in 1992, it is the agency within the U.S. Department of Health and Human Services that leads public health efforts to improve the behavioral health of the nation.

Synthetic Opioids Opioid substances that are synthesized in a laboratory and that act on the same targets in the brain and central nervous system as natural opioids (e.g., morphine and codeine).

Syringe Service Program Syringe services programs (SSPs) are community-based prevention programs that can provide linkage to substance use disorder treatment, access to and disposal of sterile syringes and injection equipment, testing, and linkage to care and treatment for infectious diseases.

T

Tapering Opioid tapering is reducing or discontinuing opioid dosage at a rate slow enough to minimize symptoms of opioid withdrawal.

The Joint Commission (TJC) An independent, not-for-profit organization, accrediting body of hospitals and healthcare organizations that provide ambulatory and office-based surgery, behavioral health, home health care, laboratory, and nursing care center services.

Tolerance Reduced response to a drug with repeated use that requires an increase in dose to achieve a similar effect.

Treatment Episode Data Set (TEDS) Supported by SAMHSA, TEDS collects demographic and drug history information about admissions and discharges to substance use disorder treatment.

U

U.S. Preventive Services Task Force (USPSTF) An independent, volunteer panel of national experts that reviews the effectiveness of disease prevention and evidence-based medicine interventions.

V

Veterans Health Administration As part of the U.S. Department of Veterans Affairs, the Veterans Health Administration is the largest integrated healthcare system in the United States, providing care at 1,255 healthcare facilities serving 9 million enrolled Veterans each year.

W

Withdrawal Management The intentional, usually medically supervised process of monitoring and managing symptoms associated with the body's reaction to a lack of opioids. Medications and devices can help suppress withdrawal symptoms during withdrawal.

World Health Organization (WHO) Founded in 1948, WHO works with 194 Member States, to provide leadership on global health matters, shape priorities, and to reinforce evidence-based standards and policies.

Index

Note: Page numbers followed by *e*, *f* and *t* indicate exhibit, figures and tables, respectively.